CURRENT CLINICAL STRATEGIES

MEDICINE

1996 Edition

Paul D. Chan, M.D.

Michael Safani, Pharm. D.
Assistant Clinical Professor
School of Pharmacy
University of California, San Francisco

Peter J. Winkle, M.D.

Preface

Current Clinical Strategies provides a link between the current medical literature and the hospital wards. For each disease entity covered, the special nursing orders, diagnostic tests, and therapeutic alternatives are presented. It is the most current source for therapeutic strategies available, including up-to-the-minute information on the treatment of AIDS and other modern diseases. This reference provides help for physicians and medical students who would like to write comprehensive admitting orders; it prevents omission of important laboratory tests and therapeutic measures.

This manual is structured to allow the clinician to individualize patient care by selecting diagnostic tests based upon clinical indications, and then to choose the clinically indicated treatment plan from the alternatives provided. Some of the specific orders may not be appropriate for a given patient, and the physician should use his or her own judgement to select orders as required by the clinical picture.

Readers are encouraged to make suggestions by writing to the publisher. Contributors will be acknowledged.

Current Clinical Strategies Publishing
9550 Warner Ave, Suite 213
Fountain Valley, California USA 92708-2822
Phone: 714-965-9400 Fax: 714-965-9401
E-Mail: 102044.2455@compuserve.com

Printed in USA   ISBN 1-881528-32-4

CONTENTS

CARDIOLOGY 6
  ADVANCED CARDIAC LIFE SUPPORT 6
  MYOCARDIAL INFARCTION & UNSTABLE ANGINA 16
  PHARMACOLOGY OF UNSTABLE ANGINA 18
  CONGESTIVE HEART FAILURE 19
  PAROXYSMAL SUPRAVENTRICULAR TACHYCARDIA 20
  VENTRICULAR ARRHYTHMIAS 21
  TORSADES DE POINTES VENTRICULAR TACHYCARDIA 21
  HYPERTENSIVE EMERGENCIES 23
  SYNCOPE 24

PULMONOLOGY 25
  ASTHMA 25
  CHRONIC OBSTRUCTIVE PULMONARY DISEASE 26
  HEMOPTYSIS 27
  ANAPHYLAXIS 28
  PLEURAL EFFUSION 29

HEMATOLOGY 31
  ANTICOAGULANT OVERDOSE 31
  DEEP VEIN THROMBOSIS 31
  PULMONARY EMBOLISM 32
  SICKLE CELL CRISIS 33

INFECTIOUS DISEASES 35
  EMPIRIC THERAPY OF MENINGITIS 35
  ENDOCARDITIS 36
  EMPIRIC THERAPY OF PNEUMONIA 38
  SPECIFIC THERAPY OF PNEUMONIA 40
  PNEUMOCYSTIS PNEUMONIA IN HIV INFECTED PATIENTS 41
  OPPORTUNISTIC INFECTIONS IN HIV INFECTED PATIENTS 42
  SEPTIC ARTHRITIS 44
  SEPTIC SHOCK 45
  CANDIDA SEPTICEMIA 46
  PERITONITIS 47
  PARACENTESIS 48
  DIVERTICULITIS 48
  LOWER URINARY TRACT INFECTION 49
  CANDIDA CYSTITIS 50
  PYELONEPHRITIS 50
  OSTEOMYELITIS 51
  TUBERCULOSIS 52
  CELLULITIS 53
  PELVIC INFLAMMATORY DISEASE 54
  NEUTROPENIC FEVER 54

GASTROENTEROLOGY 56
   PEPTIC ULCER DISEASE 56
   GASTROINTESTINAL BLEEDING 57
   CIRRHOTIC ASCITES & EDEMA 58
   VIRAL HEPATITIS 59
   CHOLECYSTITIS 60
   CHOLANGITIS & BILIARY SEPSIS 61
   PANCREATITIS 61
   EMPIRIC THERAPY OF DIARRHEA 62
   SPECIFIC THERAPY OF DIARRHEA 63
   ANTIBIOTIC ASSOCIATED & PSEUDOMEMBRANOUS COLITIS . . . 63
   CROHN'S DISEASE 64
   ULCERATIVE COLITIS 65
   PARENTERAL NUTRITION 66
   ENTERAL NUTRITION 67
   HEPATIC ENCEPHALOPATHY 68
   ALCOHOL WITHDRAWAL 69

TOXICOLOGY 70
   POISONING & DRUG OVERDOSE 70
   NARCOTIC OR PROPOXYPHENE OVERDOSE 70
   METHANOL OR ETHYLENE GLYCOL OVERDOSE 70
   CARBON MONOXIDE OVERDOSE 70
   PHENOTHIAZINE OR EXTRAPYRAMIDAL REACTION 70
   BENZODIAZEPINE OVERDOSE 70
   ACETAMINOPHEN OVERDOSE 71
   THEOPHYLLINE OVERDOSE 72
   TRICYCLIC ANTIDEPRESSANT OVERDOSE 72

NEUROLOGY 74
   ISCHEMIC STROKE 74
   TRANSIENT ISCHEMIC ATTACK 75
   SUBARACHNOID HEMORRHAGE 76
   INCREASED INTRACRANIAL PRESSURE . . . . . . : 76
   SEIZURE & STATUS EPILEPTICUS 77

ENDOCRINOLOGY 80
   DIABETIC KETOACIDOSIS 80
   NONKETOTIC HYPEROSMOLAR SYNDROME 81
   THYROTOXICOSIS 81
   HYPERTHYROIDISM 81
   MYXEDEMA COMA 82
   HYPOTHYROIDISM 82

NEPHROLOGY 84
   RENAL FAILURE 84

NEPHROLITHIASIS 85
HYPERCALCEMIA 86
HYPOCALCEMIA 86
HYPERKALEMIA 87
HYPOKALEMIA 88
HYPERMAGNESEMIA 89
HYPOMAGNESEMIA 89
HYPERNATREMIA 90
HYPONATREMIA 91
HYPERPHOSPHATEMIA 92
HYPOPHOSPHATEMIA 92

RHEUMATOLOGY 94
SYSTEMIC LUPUS ERYTHEMATOSUS 94
GOUT ATTACK 95

FORMULAS 96
DRUG LEVELS OF COMMON MEDICATIONS 97

CARDIOLOGY

ADVANCED CARDIAC LIFE SUPPORT

ALGORITHM FOR EMERGENCY CARDIAC CARE

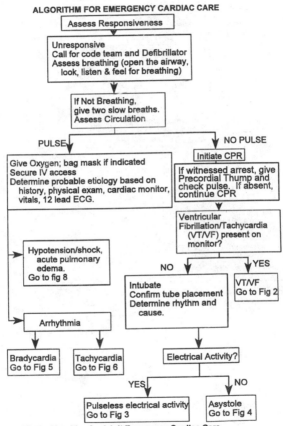

Fig 1 - Algorithm for Adult Emergency Cardiac Care

**ALGORITHM FOR VENTRICULAR FIBRILLATION AND
PULSELESS VENTRICULAR TACHYCARDIA**

Assess Airway, Breathing, Circulation
Administer CPR until defibrillator ready (precordial thump f witnessed arrest)
Ventricular Fibrillation or Tachycardia present on defibrillator

Defibrillate immediately up to 3 times at 200 J, 200-300 J, 360 J.
Do not delay defibrillation

Check pulse and Rhythm

Continue CPR
Secure IV access
Intubate if no response

Persistent or recurrent VF/VT

Return of spontaneous circulation

Pulseless Electrical Activity
Go to Fig 3

Asystole
Go to Fig 4

Continue CPR
Intubate at once
Secure IV access

Assess vital signs
Support airway
Support breathing
Provide medications appropriate for blood
    pressure, heart rate, and rhythm

Epinephrine 1 mg
IV push, repeat
q3-5min or 2 mg in
10 ml NS via ET tube
q3-5min **or**
High dose Epinephrine
0.1 mg/kg IV push,
repeat q3-5min
Defibrillate 360 J

Lidocaine 1.5 mg/kg (100 mg) IV bolus repeat q3-5min to total
loading dose of 3 mg/kg or dilute in 10 ml NS via ET tube

CPR for 30-60 sec
Defibrillate 360 J, 30-60 seconds after each dose of medication.
Repeat the pattern of drug-shock, drug-shock

Repeat Lidocaine q3-5 min OR
Bretylium 10 mg/kg IV bolus q5-10min until max 30 mg/kg.
CPR for 30-60 sec
Defibrillate 360 J

Consider Procainamide 1 gm IV over 30 min, then 1-4 mg/min.
Consider magnesium sulfate 1-2 gm IV if Torsade de Pointes, suspected
    hypomagnesemia, or severe refractory VF.
Consider Sodium Bicarbonate 1 mEq/kg IV if long arrest period or hyperkalemia.
Repeat pattern of drug-shock, drug-shock

Note: Epinephrine, lidocaine, atropine may be given via endotracheal tube at
2-2.5 times the IV dose. Dilute in 10 cc of saline.
After each intravenous dose, give 20-30 mL bolus of IV fluid &
    elevate extremity.

Fig 2 - Ventricular Fibrillation & Pulseless Ventricular Tachycardia

ALGORITHM FOR PULSELESS ELECTRICAL ACTIVITY

Pulseless Electrical Activity Includes:
 Electromechanical dissociation (EMD)
 Pseudo-EMD
 Idioventricular rhythms
 Ventricular escape rhythms
 Bradyasystolic rhythms
 Postdefibrillation idioventricular rhythms

Initiate CPR, secure IV access, intubate, assess pulse.
Doppler ultrasound assessment of blood flow may be useful

↓

Consider possible causes, and treat appropriately:
 Hypoxia (ventilate)
 Hypovolemia (infuse volume)
 Pericardial tamponade (pericardiocentesis)
 Tension pneumothorax (needle decompression)
 Pulmonary embolism (thrombectomy, thrombolytics)
 Drug overdose with tricyclics, digoxin, beta or calcium blockers
 Hyperkalemia or hypokalemia
 Acidosis (bicarbonate)
 Myocardial infarction (thrombolytics)
 Hypothemia (active rewarming)

↓

Epinephrine 1.0 mg IV bolus q3-5 min or high dose
 epinephrine 0.1 mg/kg IV push q3-5 min; may give via
 ET tube.
Continue CPR

↓

If absolute bradycardia (<60 beats/min) or relative
 bradycardia, give atroprine 1 mg IV, q3-5 min, up to total
 of 0.04 mg/kg
Consider bicarbonate, 1 mEq/kg IV (1-2 amp, 44 mEq/amp),
 if hyperkalemia or other indications.

Fig 3 - Pulseless Electrical Activity

ALGORITHM FOR ASYSTOLE

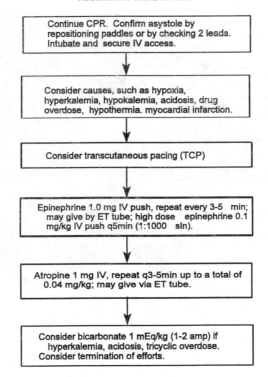

Continue CPR. Confirm asystole by repositioning paddles or by checking 2 leads. Intubate and secure IV access.

Consider causes, such as hypoxia, hyperkalemia, hypokalemia, acidosis, drug overdose, hypothermia. myocardial infarction.

Consider transcutaneous pacing (TCP)

Epinephrine 1.0 mg IV push, repeat every 3-5 min; may give by ET tube; high dose epinephrine 0.1 mg/kg IV push q5min (1:1000 sln).

Atropine 1 mg IV, repeat q3-5min up to a total of 0.04 mg/kg; may give via ET tube.

Consider bicarbonate 1 mEq/kg (1-2 amp) if hyperkalemia, acidosis, tricyclic overdose. Consider termination of efforts.

Fig 4 - Asystole

ALGORITHM FOR BRADYCARDIA

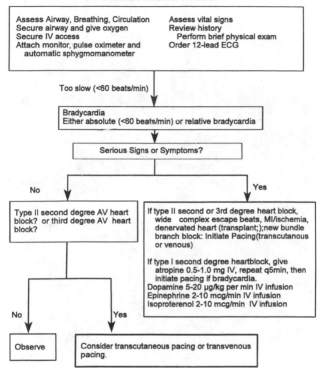

Assess Airway, Breathing, Circulation
Secure airway and give oxygen
Secure IV access
Attach monitor, pulse oximeter and
    automatic sphygmomanometer

Assess vital signs
Review history
    Perform brief physical exam
Order 12-lead ECG

Too slow (<60 beats/min)

Bradycardia
Either absolute (<60 beats/min) or relative bradycardia

Serious Signs or Symptoms?

No

Yes

Type II second degree AV heart
block? or third degree AV heart
block?

If type II second or 3rd degree heart block,
wide   complex escape beats, MI/ischemia,
denervated heart (transplant;);new bundle
branch block: Initiate Pacing(transcutaneous
or venous)

If type I second degree heartblock, give
    atropine 0.5-1.0 mg IV, repeat q5min, then
    initiate pacing if bradycardia.
Dopamine 5-20 µg/kg per min IV infusion
Epinephrine 2-10 mcg/min IV infusion
Isoproterenol 2-10 mcg/min IV infusion

No

Yes

Observe

Consider transcutaneous pacing or transvenous
pacing.

Fig 5 - Bradycardia (with patient not in cardiac arrest).

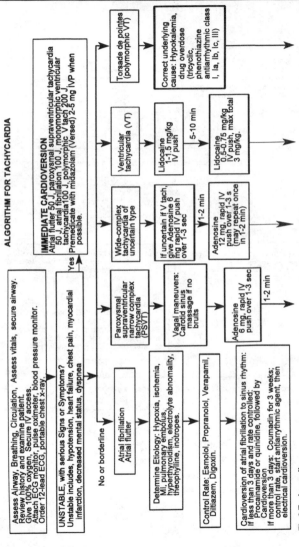

ALGORITHM FOR TACHYCARDIA

Assess Airway, Breathing, Circulation, Assess vitals, secure airway. Review history and examine patient. Give 100% oxygen, secure IV access. Attach ECG monitor, pulse oximeter, blood pressure monitor. Order 12-lead ECG, portable chest x-ray.

UNSTABLE, with serious Signs or Symptoms? Unstable includes, hypotension, heart failure, chest pain, myocardial infarction, decreased mental status, dyspnea

No or borderline

Yes →

IMMEDIATE CARDIOVERSION
Atrial flutter 50 J, paroxysmal supraventricular tachycardia 50 J, atrial fibrillation 100 J, monomorphic ventricular tachycardia 100 J, polymorphic V tach 200 J. Premedicate with midazolam (Versed) 2-5 mg IVP when possible.

No or borderline branch:

Atrial fibrillation / Atrial flutter

Determine Etiology: Hypoxia, ischemia, MI, pulmonary embolus, hyperthyroidism, electrolyte abnormality, theophylline, inotropes.

Control Rate: Esmolol, Propranolol, Verapamil, Diltiazem, Digoxin.

Cardioversion of atrial fibrillation to sinus rhythm: If less than 3 days and rate controlled; Procainamide or quinidine, followed by Cardioversion. If more than 3 days: Coumadin for 3 weeks; control rate, start antiarrhythmic agent, then electrical cardioversion.

Paroxysmal supraventricular narrow complex tachycardia (PSVT)

Vagal maneuvers: Carotid sinus massage if no bruits

Adenosine 6 mg, rapid IV push over 1-3 sec — 1-2 min →

Yes (cardioversion) branch:

Wide-complex tachycardia of uncertain type

If uncertain if V tach, give Adenosine 6 mg rapid IV push over 1-3 sec

Adenosine 12 mg, rapid IV push over 1-3 s (may repeat once in 1-2 min) — 1-2 min →

Ventricular tachycardia (VT)

Lidocaine 1-1.5 mg/kg IV push — 5-10 min

Lidocaine 0.5-0.75 mg/kg IV push, max total 3 mg/kg. →

Torsade de pointes (polymorphic VT)

Correct underlying cause: Hypokalemia, drug overdose (tricyclic, phenothiazine antiarrhythmic class I, Ia, Ib, Ic, III) →

Fig 6 Tachycardia

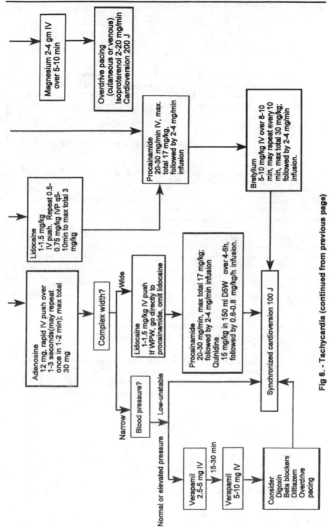

Fig 6. - Tachycardia (continued from previous page)

ALGORITHM FOR STABLE TACHYCARDIA

Stable tachycardia with serious signs and symptoms related to the tachycardia. Patient not in cardiac arrest.

If ventricular rate is >150 beats/min, prepare for immediate cardioversion. Immediate cardioversion is generally not needed for rates <150 beats/min. **Treatment of Stable Patients is based on Arrhythmia Type:**

V-Tach: Lidocaine 1-1.5 mg/kg IVP, then 0.5-0.75 mg/kg q5-10min to max total 3 mg/kg. If no response, give Procainamide 20-30 mg/min to max total 17 mg/kg, or Bretylium 5-10 mg/kg over 8-10minutes,q10min to max total 30 mg/kg.

Paroxysmal Supraventricular Tachycardia: Carotid sinus pressure if bruits absent, then adenosine 6 mg rapid IVP, followed by 12 mg rapid IVP x 2 doses to max total 30 mg. If no response, verapamil 2.5-5.0 mg IVP; may repeat dose with 5-10 mg IVP if adequate blood pressure; or Esmolol 500 mcg/kg IV over 1 min, then 50 mcg/kg/min IV infusion, and titrate up to 200 mcg/kg/min IV infusion.

Atrial Fibrillation/Flutter: Digoxin 0.5 mg IVP followed by 0.25 mg IVP q4h x 2-4 doses for rate control, then procainamide 20-30 mg/min IV to total max 17 mg/kg, followed by 2-4 mg/min IV infusion; or quinaglute 15 mg/kg IV over 4-6h, followed by 0.6-0.8 mg/kg/h IV infusion **OR** Diltiazem 0.25 mg/kg IV over 2 min, then 5-15 mg/h IV infusion.

Check Oxygen saturation, Suction device, Intubation equipment. Secure IV access

Premedicate whenever possible with Midazolam (Versed) 2-5 mg IVP or sodium pentothal 2 mg/kg rapid IVP

Synchronized cardioversion
Atrialflutter	50 J
PSVT	50 J
Atrial	100 J
Monomorphic V-tach	100 J
Polymorphic V tach	200 J

Fig 7 - Stable Tachycardia (not in cardiac arrest)

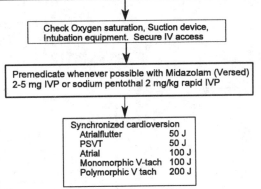

ALGORITHM FOR HYPOTENSION, SHOCK, AND ACUTE PULMONARY EDEMA

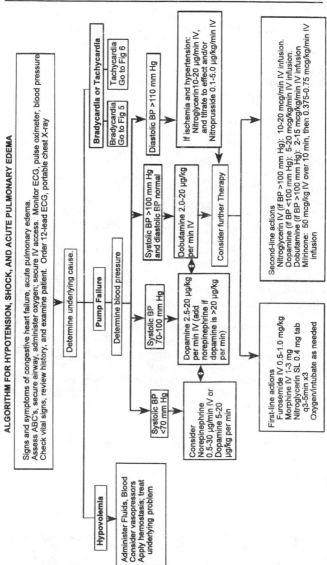

Signs and symptoms of congestive heart failure, acute pulmonary edema.
Assess ABC's, secure airway, administer oxygen; secure IV access. Monitor ECG, pulse oximeter, blood pressure
Check vital signs, review history, and examine patient. Order 12-lead ECG, portable chest X-ray

Determine underlying cause.

Hypovolemia

Administer Fluids, Blood
Consider vasopressors
Apply hemostasis; treat
underlying problem

Pump Failure

Determine blood pressure

Systolic BP <70 mm Hg

Consider
Norepinephrine
0.5-30 µg/min IV or
Dopamine 5-20
µg/kg per min

Systolic BP 70-100 mm Hg

Dopamine 2.5-20 µg/kg
per min IV (add
norepinephrine if
dopamine is >20 µg/kg
per min)

Systolic BP >100 mm Hg
and diastolic BP normal

Dobutamine 2.0-20 µg/kg
per min IV

Consider further Therapy

Bradycardia or Tachycardia

Bradycardia
Go to Fig 5

Tachycardia
Go to Fig 6

Diastolic BP >110 mm Hg

If ischemia and hypertension:
Nitroglycerin 10-20 µg/min IV,
and titrate to effect and/or
Nitroprusside 0.1-5.0 µg/kg/min IV

First-line actions
Furosemide IV 0.5-1.0 mg/kg
Morphine IV 1-3 mg
Nitroglycerin SL 0.4 mg tab
q3-5min x3
Oxygen/intubate as needed

Second-line actions
Nitroglycerin IV (if BP >100 mm Hg): 10-20 mcg/kg/min IV infusion.
Dopamine (if BP <100 mm Hg): 5-20 mcg/kg/min IV infusion
Dobutamine (if BP >100 mm Hg): 2-15 mcg/kg/min IV infusion
Milrinone: 50 mcg/kg IV over 10 min, then 0.375-0.75 mg/kg/min IV
infusion

Fig 8 - Hypotension, Shock, and Acute Pulmonary Edema.

MYOCARDIAL INFARCTION & UNSTABLE ANGINA

1. **Admit to:** Monitored bed (CCU/MICU)
2. **Diagnosis:** Chest pain/rule out MI
3 **Condition:**
4. **Vital signs:** q1h, then q6h. Call physician if pulse >90,<60; BP >150/90, <90/60; R>25, <12; T >38.5°C.
5. **Activity:** Bed rest with bedside commode.
7. **Nursing:** Guaiac stools. If patient has chest pain, obtain 12-lead ECG and call physician.
8. **Diet:** Cardiac diet, 1-2 gm sodium, low fat, low cholesterol diet. No caffeine or temperature extremes.
9. **IV Fluids:** D5W at TKO
10. **Special Medications:**
  -Oxygen 2-4 L/min by NC.
  -Aspirin 80 or 325 mg PO chew and swallow, then aspirin E.C. (Ecotrin)160 or 325 mg PO qd.
  -Nitroglycerine Drip 15 mcg IV bolus, then 10 mcg/min infusion (50 mg in 250-500 mL D5W, 100-200 mcg/mL). Titrate in 5-10 mcg/min steps, up to 200-300 mcg/min; maintain systolic BP >90; titrate to control symptoms; keep heart rate <20% of baseline rate **OR**
  -Nitroglycerine SL, 0.4 mg (0.15-0.6 mg) SL q5min until pain free (up to 3 tabs)

Thrombolytic Therapy in Myocardial Infarction:
Relative Contraindications to Thrombolytics: Absence of ST-segment elevation, severe hypertension, cerebrovascular disease, relatively recent surgery (>2 wk), cardiopulmonary resuscitation.
Absolute Contraindications to Thrombolytics: Active internal bleeding, history of hemorrhagic stroke, head trauma, pregnancy, surgery within 2 wk, recent non-compressible vascular puncture.

A. Streptokinase or Anistreplase (APSAC):
1. Aspirin 325 mg chew and swallow now and qd **AND**
   Heparin 5000 U IV bolus **AND**
   Diphenhydramine 50 mg IV push **AND**
   Methylprednisolone 250 mg IV push.
2. Streptokinase - 1.5 million IU of streptokinase in 100 mL NS IV over 60 min **OR**
   Anistreplase (APSAC, Eminase), 30 units IV over 2-5min.
3. Heparin 10 U/kg/h IV after administration of streptokinase or anistreplase and maintain PTT 1.5-2 times control.
4. PTT, fibrinogen now **AND** q6h x 24h.
5. No IM or arterial punctures, watch IV for bleeding.

OR

B. Recombinant tissue plasminogen activator (tPA):

1. Aspirin, 325 mg chew and swallow now & qd. Heparin 5000 U IV bolus.
2. tPA 15 mg IVP over 2 min, followed by 0.75 mg/kg (max 50 mg) IV infusion over 30 min, followed by 0.5 mg/kg (max 35 mg) IV infusion over 60 min (total dose $\leq$ 100 mg).
3. Start heparin 15 U/kg/h infusion after tPA, & adjust to PTT of 1.5-2 times control.
4. PTT & fibrinogen now & q6h x 24h. No IM or arterial punctures, watch IV for bleeding.
5. **Labs:** INR/PTT, thrombin time, FDP, fibrinogen, reptilase time, bleed time, type & screen.

Beta-Blockers: Contraindicated in presence of CHF.

-Metoprolol (Lopressor) 5 mg IV q2-5min x 3 doses; then 25 mg PO q6h x 48h, then 100 mg PO q12h; may give 2 mg IV q2h prn pulse > 70, hold if systolic BP <90 **OR**

-Esmolol hydrochloride (Brevibloc) 500 mcg/kg IV over 1 min, then 50 mcg/kg/min IV infusion, titrated to heart rate <60 (max 300 mcg/kg/min) **OR**

-Propranolol 0.1 mg/kg IV divided in 3 doses q5min; followed in 1h by 20-40 mg PO q6-8h (160-240 mg/d); propranolol-LA (Inderal-LA), 80-120 mg PO qd [60, 80, 120, 160 mg] **OR**

-Atenolol (Tenormin) 5-10 mg IV, then 50-100 mg PO qd, titrate to HR <60 (max 200 mg/d).

Other Medications

-Heparin 5000 U (100 U/kg) IV bolus followed by 1000 U/hr (15 U/kg); adjust to PTT 2-2.5 times control **OR** 5000 units SQ q8-12h.

-Isosorbide dinitrate (Isordil) 10-60 mg PO tid [5,10,20, 30,40 mg]; Sustained release, 40-80 mg PO q8-12h [40 mg]

11. Symptomatic Medications:

-Acetaminophen (Tylenol) 325-650 mg PO q4-6h prn headache.

-Lorazepam (Ativan) 1-2 mg PO tid or qid prn anxiety **OR**

-Zolpidem (Ambien) 5-10 mg qhs, use 5 mg for elderly **OR**

-Diphenhydramine (Benadryl) 25-50 mg PO qhs prn sleep.

-Docusate (Colace) 100-250 mg PO bid.

-Dimenhydrinate (Dramamine) 25-50 mg IV over 2-5 min q4-6h or 50 mg PO q4-6h prn nausea.

-Ranitidine (Zantac) 150 mg PO bid or 50 mg IV q8h.

-Mylanta 30 mL PO qid prn heartburn.

12. Extras: ECG stat and in 12h and in AM. Repeat if chest pain; portable CXR, echocardiogram or radionuclide ventriculogram. Cardiology consult.

13. Labs: SMA7 & 12, magnesium. Cardiac enzymes: CPK, CPK-MB, STAT & q6h x 24h. LDH & isoenzymes. CBC; fasting cholesterol, HDL, triglyceride. INR/PTT, UA.

14. Other Orders and Meds:

_____

PHARMACOLOGY OF UNSTABLE ANGINA

	Benefits			
Drug	Reduce Mortality	Prevent AMI	Reduce Angina	Disadvantages
Aspirin	+++	+++	---	Bleeding
Heparin	---	+++	++	Bleeding, thrombocytopenia
Nitrates	---	+	+++	Tolerance, hypotension
Beta blockers	---	+	+++	Bronchoconstriction, AV block, reduced contractility
Calcium blockers	---	---	+++	Hypotension, AV block, reduced contractility, tachycardia.
Lytic therapy	---	---	+	bleeding

AMI = acute myocardial infarction; AV = atrioventricular
Rutherford JD, et al. Pharmacology of Angina. Am J Cardiol 1993; 72: 16 C-20 C

CONGESTIVE HEART FAILURE

1. **Admit to:**
2. **Diagnosis:** Congestive Heart Failure
3. **Condition:**
4. **Vital signs:** q1h. Call physician if P>120; BP >150/100 <80/60; T >38.5°C; R >25 <10.
5. **Activity:** Bed rest with bedside commode.
6. **Nursing:** Daily weights, measure inputs and outputs, Head of bed at 45 degrees, legs elevated.
7. **Diet:** 1-2 gm salt, cardiac diet. Fluid intake of 1.5 L/d.
8. **IV Fluids:** Hep-lock with flush q shift.
9. **Special Medications:**
   -Oxygen 2-4 L/min by NC.

Diuretics:
-Furosemide 10-160 mg IV qd or 20-80 mg PO qAM [20,40,80 mg] **OR**
-Bumetanide (Bumex) 0.5-1 mg IV q2-3h until response; then 0.5-1.0 mg IV q8-24h (max 10 mg/d); or 0.5-2.0 mg PO qAM **OR**
-Metolazone (Zaroxolyn) 2.5-10 mg PO qd, max 20 mg/d; 30 min before loop diuretic [2.5,5,10 mg].

Digoxin:
-Digoxin Maintenance - 0.125-0.5 mg PO or IV qd [0.125,0.25, 0.5 mg].

Angiotensin- II Receptor Antagonist:
-Losartan (Cozaar) 25-50 mg PO qd-bid, max 100 mg/day [25, 50 mg]; does not cause cough or angioedema.

ACE Inhibitors:
-Quinapril (Accupril) Initially 5-10 mg PO qd, then 20-80 mg PO qd in 1 to 2 divided doses [5,10,20,40 mg].
-Lisinopril (Zestril, Prinivil) 5-40 mg PO qd [5,10,20,40 mg].
-Benazepril (Lotensin) 10-40 mg PO qd, max 80 mg/d [5,10,20,40 mg].
-Fosinopril (Monopril) 10-40 mg PO qd, max 80 mg/d [10,20 mg].
-Ramipril (Altace) 2.5-10 mg PO qd, max 20 mg/d [1.25,2.5,5,10 mg].
-Captopril (Capoten) 6.25-50 mg PO q8h [12.5, 25,50,100 mg] **OR**
-Enalapril (Vasotec) 1.25-5 mg slow IV push q6h or 2.5-20 mg PO bid [5,10,20 mg] **OR**

Inotropic Agents:
-Dopamine 3-15 mcg/kg/min IV (400 mg in 250 cc D5W, 1600 mcg/mL), titrate to CO >4, CI >2; systolic > 90 **AND/OR**
-Dobutamine 2.5-10 mcg/kg/min, max of 14 mcg/kg/min (500 mg in 250 mL D5W, 2 mcg/mL) **AND/OR**
-Milrinone (Primacor) 50 mcg/kg IV over 10 min, followed by 0.375-0.75 (average 0.5) mcg/kg/min IV infusion (40 mg in 200 mLs NS (QS), conc=0.2 mg/mL).

Nitrates and Nitroprusside:
   -Nitroglycerine 10 mcg/min IV (50 mg in 250-500 mL D5W) **OR**
   -Isosorbide dinitrate (Isordil) 40 mg PO qid.

Other Agents and Potassium:
   -KCL (Micro-K) 20-60 mEq PO qd.

10. Symptomatic Medications:
   -Heparin 5000 U SQ q12h.
   -Docusate sodium 100-200 mg PO qhs.
   -Ranitidine (Zantac)150 mg PO bid or 50 mg IV q8h.

11. Extras: CXR PA & LAT, ECG now & repeat if chest pain or palpitations, echocardiogram, radionuclide ventriculogram.

12. Labs: SMA 7 & 12, albumin, CBC; cardiac enzymes: CPK, CPK-MB, STAT & q6h x 24h. Thyroid stimulating hormone and free thyroxine. Repeat SMA 7 in AM. Digoxin level. UA.

13. Other orders and meds:

PAROXYSMAL SUPRAVENTRICULAR TACHYCARDIA

1. **Admit to:**
2. **Diagnosis:** PSVT
3. **Condition:**
4. **Vital signs:** q1h. Call physician if BP >160/90, <90/60; apical pulse >130, <50; R >25, <10; T >38.5°C
5. **Activity:** Bedrest with bedside commode.
6. **Nursing:**
7. **Diet:** Low fat, low cholesterol, no caffeine.
8. **IV Fluids:** D5W at TKO.
9. **Special Medications:**

Attempt vagal maneuvers (Valsalva maneuver and/or carotid sinus massage)
   before drug therapy (If no bruits).

Cardioversion (if unstable or refractory to drug therapy):
   1. NPO x 6h, dig level ≤2.4 & potassium must be normal.
   2. Midazolam (Versed) 2.5 mg IV.
   3. If stable, cardiovert with synchronized 10-50 J, increase by 50 J increments. If unstable, start with 75-100 J, then increase to 200 J and 360 J.

Pharmacologic Therapy of PSVT:
   -Adenosine (Adenocard) 6 mg rapid IV over 1-2 sec, followed by saline flush, may repeat 12 mg IV after 2-3 min, up to max of 30 mg total (ineffective if on theophylline) **OR**
   -Verapamil (Isoptin) 2.5-10 mg IV over 2-3min (may give calcium gluconate 1 gm IV over 3-6 min prior to verapamil); then 40-120 mg PO q8h or verapamil SR 120-240 mg PO qd **OR**

-Esmolol hydrochloride (Brevibloc) 500 mcg/kg IV over 1 min, then 50 mcg/kg/min IV infusion titrated to HR of <60 (max of 300 mcg/kg/min) **OR**

-Diltiazem (Cardizem) 0.25 mg/kg (ave 20 mg) IV over 2 min, then 5-15 mg/hr IV infusion [100 mg/D5W 250 mLs (QS); conc 0.4 mg/mL]. For control of ventricular response rate only in atrial fibrillation/flutter.

-Propranolol 1-5 mg (0.15 mg/kg) given IV in 1 mg aliquots min; then 60-80 mg PO tid; propranolol-LA (Inderal-LA), 80-120 mg PO qd [60, 80, 120, 160 mg] **OR**

-Digoxin aliquots of 0.25 mg q4h as needed; then 0.125-0.25 mg PO or IV qd **OR**

10.Symptomatic Medications:

-Lorazepam (Ativan) 1-2 mg PO tid prn anxiety.

11.Extras: Portable CXR, ECG; repeat if chest pain. Cardiology consult.

12.Labs: CBC, SMA 7 & 12, Mg, thyroid panel. Drug levels, toxicology screen, UA.

13. Other Orders and Meds:

Differential Points Distinguishing Supraventricular Tachycardia (SVT) from Aberrancy from Ventricular Tachycardia (VT)

	VT	SVT w/aberrancy
QRS width	>0.14 sec	<0.14 sec
Axis	Left or bizarre	Normal
V_1	Rs, Rsr', RsR'	rsR'
V_6	S wave present	S wave absent
Fusion beats	Present	Absent
Atrioventricular dissociation	Present	Absent

VENTRICULAR ARRHYTHMIAS

1. Ventricular Fibrillation & Tachycardia:

-**If unstable (see ACLS protocol page 6):** Defibrillate with unsynchronized 200 J, then 300 J.

-Oxygen 100% by mask.

-Lidocaine loading dose 75-100 mg IV, then 2-4 mg/min IV **OR**

-Procainamide loading dose 10-15 mg/kg at 20 mg/min IV or 100 mg IV q5min, then 1-4 mg/min IV maintenance **OR**

-Bretylium loading dose 5-10 mg/kg over 5-10 min, then 1-4 mg/min IV.

-**Also see "other antiarrhythmics" below.**

2. TORSADES DE POINTES VENTRICULAR TACHYCARDIA:

-Correct underlying cause & consider discontinuing quinidine, procainamide, disopyramide, moricizine, lidocaine, amiodarone, phenothiazine, haloperidol, tricyclic and tetracyclic antidepressants, ketoconazole, itraconazole, terfenadine, astemizole, bepridil, hypokalemia, and hypomagnesemia.

-Magnesium sulfate (drug of choice) 1-4 gm in IV bolus over 5-15 min or infuse 3-20 mg/min for 7-48h until QT interval <0.5 sec.

-Isoproterenol (Isuprel), 2-20 mcg/min (2 mg in 500 mL D5W, 4 mcg/mL) **OR**

-Phenytoin (Dilantin) 100-300 mg IV given in 50 mg aliquots q5min.

-Consider ventricular pacing and/or cardioversion.

3. Other Antiarrhythmics:

Class I:

-Moricizine (Ethmozine) 200-300 mg PO q8h, max 900 mg/d.

Class Ia:

-Quinidine sulfate 200-600 mg PO q4-6h (max 2.4 gm/d) or gluconate 324-648 mg PO q8-12h **OR**

-Procainamide PO loading dose of 750-1000 mg (15 mg/kg) in 2-3 divided doses, then 250-1000 mg PO q4-6h or 1 gm IV load given as 100 mg IV q5min or 20 mg/min until arrhythmia suppressed, then 2-6 mg/min IV infusion **OR**

-Disopyramide 100-300 mg PO q6-8h.

Class Ib:

-Lidocaine 75-100 mg IV, then 2-4 mg/min IV **OR**

-Mexiletine (Mexitil) 100-200 mg PO q8h, max 1200 mg/d **OR**

-Tocainide (Tonocard) loading 400-600 mg PO, then 400-600 mg PO q8-12h (1200-1800 mg/d PO in divided doses q8-12h **OR**

-Phenytoin, loading dose 100-300 mg IV given as 50 mg in NS over 10 min IV q5min, then 100 mg IV q5min prn.

Class Ic:

-Flecainide (Tambocor) 50-100 mg PO q12h, max 400 mg/d.

-Propafenone (Rythmol) 150-300 mg PO q8h, max 1200 mg/d.

Class II:

-Propranolol 1-3 mg IV in NS (max 0.15 mg/kg) or 20-80 mg PO q6h (80-160 mg/d); propranolol-LA (Inderal-LA), 80-120 mg PO qd [60, 80, 120, 160 mg] **OR**

-Esmolol loading dose 500 mcg/kg over 1 min, then 50-200 mcg/kg/min IV infusion **OR**

-Atenolol 50-100 mg/d PO **OR**

-Nadolol 40-100 mg PO qd-bid **OR**

-Metoprolol 50-100 mg PO bid-tid **OR**

-Timolol 20 mg/d PO.

Class III:

-Amiodarone (Cordarone) PO loading 400-1200 mg/d in divided doses x 5-14 days, then 200-400 mg PO qd (5-10 mg/kg) **OR**

-Bretylium 5-10 mg/kg IV over 5-10 min, then maintenance of 1-4 mg/min IV or repeat boluses 5-10 mg/kg IV q6-8h; infusion of 1-4 mg/min IV.

-Sotalol (Betapace) 40-80 mg PO bid, max 320 mg/d in 2-3 divided doses.
4. **Extras:** CXR, ECG, echocardiogram, Holter monitor, signal averaged ECG, cardiology consult.
5. **Labs:** SMA 7&12, Mg, calcium, CBC, LFT's, drug levels, thyroid function test. UA.
6. **Other Orders and Meds:**

HYPERTENSIVE EMERGENCIES

1. **Admit to:**
2. **Diagnosis:** Emergencies Hypertension
3. **Condition:**
4. **Vital signs:** q30min until BP controlled, then q4h. Call physician if sudden change in BP >30 mmHg systolic; BP systolic >200, <90; diastolic >120, <60; P >120
5. **Activity:** bed rest
6. **Nursing:** Intra-arterial BP monitoring, daily weights, I&O.
7. **Diet:** Clear liquids.
8. **IV Fluids:** D5W at TKO.
9. **Special Medications:**
   -Nitroprusside sodium 0.25-10 mcg/kg/min IV (50 mg in 250 mL of D5W), titrate to desired BP. Discontinue if acute fall in BP >30 systolic **OR**
   -Nitroglycerin 5-100 mcg/min IV, titrated to desired BP, up to 300 mcg/min (50 mg in 250-500 mL D5W) **OR**
   -Labetalol (Trandate, Normodyne) 20 mg IV bolus (0.25 mg/kg), then 20-80 mg boluses IV q10-15min titrated to desired BP (max of 300 mg). Infusion of 1.0-2.0 mg/min **OR**
   -Clonidine (Catapres), initial 0.1-0.2 mg PO followed by 0.05-0.1 mg per hour until DBP <115 (max total dose of 0.8 mg); then 0.1-2.4 mg/d in divided doses bid-tid, max 2.4 mg/d. Clonidine patch (Catapres-TTS) 0.1-0.3 mg/24h apply q7 days [0.1,0.2,0.3 mg/24h] **OR**
   -Nifedipine (Procardia) 5-20 mg SL or PO (bite & swallow punctured capsule, 0.25-0.5 mg/kg/dose), repeat prn **OR**
   -Enalapril (Vasotec) 1.25-5 mg slow IV push q6h, then 2.5-20 mg PO bid **OR**
   -Phentolamine (pheochromocytoma), 5-10 mg IV, repeated as needed up to 20 mg. Monoamine oxidase inhibitor with hypertensive crisis 5 mg slow IV push q4-6h (norepinephrine at bedside to treat hypotension). **OR**
   -Trimethaphan camsylate (Arfonad)(dissecting aneurysm) 2-4 mg/min IV infusion (500 mg in 500 mL D5W).
10. **Symptomatic Medications:**
11. **Extras:** Portable CXR, ECG, echocardiogram.

12. Labs: CBC, SMA 7, UA with micro. Thyroid stimulating hormone, free T4, 24h urine for metanephrine. Plasma catecholamines, plasma renin activity. Urine drug screen.

13. Other Orders and Meds:

SYNCOPE

1. Admit to:

2. Diagnosis: Syncope

3. Condition:

4. Vital signs: q1h, postural BP & pulse q12h; Call physician if BP >160/90, <90/60; P >120, <50; R>25, <10

5. Activity: Bed rest.

6. Nursing: Fingerstick glucose.

7. Diet: Regular

8. IV Fluids: D5W at TKO.

9. Special medications:

Vasovagal Syncope:

   -Scopolamine 1.5 mg transdermal patch q3 days.

Postural Syncope:

   -Fludrocortisone 0.1-1 mg/d PO.

   -Ibuprofen 200-800 mg PO qid.

10. Extras: CXR, ECG, signal averaged ECG, 24h Holter monitor, tilt test, EEG, echocardiogram, carotid duplex scan, CT/MRI.

11. Labs: CBC, SMA 7 & 12, CPK isoenzymes, Mg, Calcium. Blood alcohol, drug levels. UA, urine drug screen.

12. Other Orders and Meds:

PULMONOLOGY

ASTHMA

1. **Admit to:**
2. **Diagnosis:** Exacerbation of asthma
3. **Condition:**
4. **Vital signs:** q6h. Call physician if P >140; R >30, <10; T >38.5°C; O2 Sat <90%
5. **Activity:**
6. **Nursing:** Peak flow rate pre & post bronchodilator treatments, pulse oximeter. Avoid aspirin containing medications and sedatives. Measure bedside peak respiratory flow q2h with portable peak flowmeter.
7. **Diet:** Regular, no caffeine.
8. **IV Fluids:** D5½NS, at 125 cc/h.
9. **Special Medications:**
   -Oxygen 2-6 L/min by NC. Keep O2 sat >90%.

Beta Agonists, Acute Treatment:
   -Albuterol (Ventolin), 0.2-0.5 mL (2.5 mg) in 3 mL saline q2-8h prn (5 mg/mL sln) **OR**
   -Albuterol (Ventolin) or Metaproterenol (Alupent) MDI 3-8 puffs, then 2 puffs q3-6h prn or powder 200 mcg/capsule inhaled qid prn.

Systemic Corticosteroids:
   -Methylprednisolone (Solu-Medrol) 60-125 mg IV q6h; then 30-60 mg PO qd. **OR**
   -Prednisone 20-60 mg PO qAM.

Aminophylline & Theophylline:
   -Aminophylline load dose: 5.6 mg/kg **total** body weight in 100 mL D5W IV over 20min. Maintenance of 0.5-0.6 mg/kg **ideal** body weight/h (500 mg in 250 mL D5W); reduce if elderly, heart/liver failure (0.2-0.4 mg/kg/hr); may need up to 0.8-0.9 mg/kg/h if smoker. Reduce load 50-75% if taking theophylline (1 mg/kg of aminophylline will raise levels 2 mcg/mL) **OR**
   -Theophylline IV solution loading dose 4.5 mg/kg **total** body weight, then 0.4-0.5 mg/kg **ideal** body weight/hr.
   -Theophylline (Theo-Dur) PO loading dose of 6 mg/kg, then maintenance of 100-400 mg PO bid-tid (3 mg/kg q8h); 80% of total daily IV aminophylline in 2-3 doses.

Inhaled Corticosteroids:
   -Beclomethasone (Beclovent)(when off IV steroids) MDI 2-6 puffs qid, with spacer 5min after bronchodilator, followed by gargling with water **OR**
   -Triamcinolone (Azmacort) MDI 1-4 puffs tid-qid **OR**
   -Flunisolide (AeroBid) MDI 2-4 puffs bid **OR**
   -Budesonide 200-800 mcg qid MDI (50 mcg/puff or 250 mcg/puff).

-After stabilization, inhaled corticosteroids should be the mainstay of treatment.

Other Beta Agonists:
-Pirbuterol (Maxair) MDI 2 puffs q4-6h **OR**
-Bitolterol (Tornalate) MDI 2-3 puffs q1-3min initially, then 2-3 puffs q4-8h **OR**
-Fenoterol (Berotec) MDI 3 puffs initially, then 2 bid-qid.

Acute Bronchitis
-Ampicillin/sulbactam (Unasyn) 1.5 gm IV q6h **OR**
-Ampicillin 0.5-1 gm IV q6h or 250-500 mg PO qid **OR**
-Cefuroxime (Zinacef) 750 mg IV q8h **OR**
-Bactrim DS, 1 tab PO bid **OR**
-Amoxicillin/clavulanate (Augmentin) 250-500 mg PO q8h **OR**
-Cefaclor (Ceclor) 250-500 mg PO q8h.

10. Symptomatic Medications:
-Docusate sodium (Colace) 100-200 mg PO qhs.
-Ranitidine (Zantac) 50 mg IV q8h or 150 mg PO bid.

11. Extras: Portable CXR, ECG, pulmonary function tests pre and post bronchodilators; pulmonary rehabilitation.

12. Labs: ABG, CBC, SMA7. Theophylline level stat & after 24h of infusion. Sputum Gram stain, C&S.

13. Other Orders and Meds:

CHRONIC OBSTRUCTIVE PULMONARY DISEASE

1. **Admit to:**
2. **Diagnosis:** Exacerbation of COPD
3. **Condition:**
4. **Vital signs:** q4h. Call physician if P >130; R >30, <10; T >38.5°C; O2 Sat <90%.
5. **Activity:** Bed rest, up in chair if able; bedside commode.
6. **Nursing:** Pulse oximeter. Measure peak flow with portable peak flowmeter bid and chart with vital signs. No sedatives.
7. **Diet:** No added salt, no caffeine. Push fluids.
8. **IV Fluids:** D5½NS with 20 mEq KCL/L at 125 cc/h.
9. **Special Medications:**
   -O2 1-2 L/min by NC or 24-35% by Venturi mask, keep O2 saturation 90-91%.

Beta Agonists, Acute Treatment:
-Nebulized Albuterol (Ventolin) 0.2-0.5 mL (2.5 mg) in 3 mL of saline q2-8h prn (5 mg/mL sln) **OR**
-Albuterol (Ventolin) or Metaproterenol (Alupent) MDI 2-4 puffs q4-6h prn.

Corticosteroids & Anticholinergics:
-Methylprednisolone (Solu-Medrol) 40-60 mg IV q6h or 30-60 mg PO qd
Followed by:
-Prednisone 40-60 mg PO qd, taper to minimum dose.
-Triamcinolone (Azmacort) MDI 2-4 puffs qid **OR**
-Beclomethasone (Beclovent) MDI 2-6 puffs qid, with spacer, 5 min after
bronchodilator, followed by gargling with water **OR**
-Flunisolide (AeroBid) MDI 2-4 puffs bid.
-Ipratropium Bromide (Atrovent) MDI 2 puffs tid-qid
Aminophylline & Theophylline:
-Aminophylline loading dose - 5.6 mg/kg **total** body weight over 20 min (if not
already on theophylline); then 0.5-0.6 mg/kg **ideal** body weight/hr (500 mg
in 250 mL of D5W at 20 cc/h); reduce if elderly, or heart or liver disease
(0.2-0.4 mg/kg/hr). Reduce loading to 50-75% if already taking theo-
phylline (1 mg/kg of aminophylline will raise levels by 2 mcg/mL) **OR**
-Theophylline IV solution loading dose, 4.5 mg/kg **total** body weight, then
0.4-0.5 mg/kg **ideal** body weight/hr.
-Theophylline long acting (Theo-Dur) PO maintenance dose of 100-400 mg
PO bid-tid (3 mg/kg q8h); 80% of daily IV aminophylline in 2-3 doses.
Acute Bronchitis
-Ampicillin 1 gm IV q6h or 250-500 mg PO qid **OR**
-Trimethoprim/Sulfamethoxazole (Septra DS) 160/800 mg PO bid or 160/800
mg IV q8-12h (10-15 mL in 100 cc D5W tid) **OR**
-Cefuroxime (Zinacef) 750 mg IV q8h **OR**
-Ampicillin/sulbactam (Unasyn) 1.5 gm IV q6h **OR**
-Cefuroxime (Ceclor) 1.5 gm IV q8h **OR**
10. Symptomatic Medications:
-Docusate sodium (Colace) 100-200 mg PO qhs.
-Ranitidine (Zantac)150 mg PO bid or 50 mg IV q8h.
11. Extras: Portable CXR, PFT's with bronchodilators, ECG.
12. Labs: ABG, CBC, SMA7. UA. Theo level stat & after 12-24h of infusion.
Sputum Gram stain & C&S; alpha 1 antitrypsin level.
13. Other Orders and Meds:

HEMOPTYSIS

1. **Admit to:**
2. **Diagnosis:** Hemoptysis
3. **Condition:**
4. **Vital signs:** q1-6h; Orthostatic BP & pulse bid. Call physician if BP >160/90,
<90/60; P >130, <50; R>25, <10; T >38.5°C; O2 sat <90%

5. **Activity:** Bed rest with bedside commode. Keep patient in lateral decubitus, Trendelenburg's position, bleeding side down.
6. **Nursing:** Quantify all sputum and expectorated blood; suction prn. O2 at 100% by mask, pulse oximeter. Discontinue narcotics & sedatives. Have double lumen endotracheal tube available for use.
7. **Diet:**
8. **IV Fluids:** NS at 0.5-1 L/hr x 1-3 L ($\geq$16 gauge), then transfuse PRBC, Foley to gravity.
9. **Special Medications:**
   -Transfuse 2-6 U PRBC over 2-6h.
10. **Other Considerations:**
    -Consider empiric antibiotics if any suggestion that bronchitis or infection may be contributing to hemoptysis.
11. **Extras:** CXR PA, LAT, ECG, VQ scan, contrast CT, bronchoscopy. PPD & controls, pulmonary & thoracic surgery consults.
12. **Labs:** Type & cross 4-6 U PRBC. ABG, CBC, platelets, SMA7 & 12, ESR. Anti-glomerular basement antibody, rheumatoid factor, complement, anti-nuclear cytoplasmic antibody. Sputum Gram stain, C&S, AFB, fungal, & cytology qAM x 3 days. UA, INR/PTT, von Willebrand Factor. Repeat CBC q6h.
13. **Other Orders and Meds:**

ANAPHYLAXIS

1. **Admit to:**
2. **Diagnosis:** Anaphylaxis
3. **Condition:**
4. **Vital signs:** q1-6h; Call physician if BP systolic >160, <90; diastolic. >90, <60; P >120, <50; R>25, <10; T >38.5°C
5. **Activity:** Bedrest
6. **Nursing:** I&O q1-6h, O2 at 6 L/min by NC or mask. Place patient in Trendelenburg's position, No. 4 or 5 endotracheal tube at bedside.
7. **Diet:** NPO
8. **IV Fluids:** 2 IV lines. Normal saline or LR 1-4 L over 1-3h, then D5½NS at 150-200 cc/h. Foley to closed drainage.
9. **Special Medications:**

Gastrointestinal Decontamination:
   -Gastric lavage if indicated for recent oral ingestion.
   -Activated charcoal 50-100 gm, followed by cathartic.

Bronchodilators:
   -Epinephrine (1:1000) 0.3-0.5 mL SQ or IM q10min or 1-4 mcg/min IV **OR** in severe life threatening reactions give 0.5 mg (5.0 mL of 1: 10,000 sln) IV q5-10min prn. **OR** dilute in 10 mL NS & give via endotracheal tube. Epi-

nephrine, 0.3 mg of 1:1000 sln may be injected SQ at site of allergen injection **OR**
-Aerosolized 2% racemic epinephrine 0.5-0.75 mL **OR**
-Albuterol (Ventolin) 0.5%, 0.5 mL in 2.5 mL NS q30min by nebulizer prn.
-Aminophylline loading dose 5.6 mg/kg **total** body weight IV, then infuse 0.3-0.9 mg/kg **ideal** body weight/h **OR**
-Theophylline IV solution, loading dose 4.5 mg/kg **total** body weight, then 0.4-0.5 mg/kg **ideal** body weight/hr.

Corticosteroids:
-Methylprednisolone (Solu-Medrol) 50 mg IV q4-6h **OR**
-Methylprednisolone acetate (Depo-Medrol) 40-80 mg IM **OR**
-Hydrocortisone Sodium Succinate 200-500 mg IV q4-6h (IV steroids should be followed by PO steroids).

Antihistamines:
-Diphenhydramine (Benadryl) 25-50 mg IV, IM or PO q2-4h **OR**
-Hydroxyzine (Vistaril) 25-50 mg IV, IM or PO q2-4h.
-Cimetidine (Tagamet) 300 mg IV or PO q6h **OR**
-Ranitidine (Zantac) 150 mg IV or PO bid.

Pressors & other Agents:
-Norepinephrine (Levophed) 8-12 mcg/min IV, adjust to systolic 100 mmHg (8 mg in 500 mL D5W) **OR**
-Isoproterenol (Isuprel) 0.5-5 mcg/min IV **OR**
-Dopamine (Intropin) 5-20 mcg/kg/min IV.

10. Extras: Portable CXR, ECG.

11. Labs: CBC, SMA 7&12; 24h urine for 5-hydroxyindoleacetic acid (carcinoid), UA.

12. Other Orders and Meds:

PLEURAL EFFUSION

1. Admit to:

2. Diagnosis: Pleural effusion

3. Condition:

4. Vital signs: q shift; Call physician if BP >160/90, <90/60; P>120, <50; R>25, <10; T >38.5°C

5. Activity:

6. Diet: Regular.

7. IV Fluids: D5W at TKO

8. Extras: CXR PA & LAT repeat after thoracentesis; bilateral lateral decubitus ECG, ultrasound; PPD with control antigens (candida, mumps); pulmon consult.

9. Labs: CBC, SMA 7 & 12, protein, albumin, amylase, rheumatoid factor, ANA, ESR, INR/PTT, UA. Fungal serologies.

Pleural fluid:

<u>**Tube 1**</u> - LDH, protein, amylase, triglyceride, glucose (10 mL).

<u>**Tube 2**</u> - Gram stain, C&S, AFB, fungal C&S (20-60 mL, heparinized).

<u>**Tube 3**</u> - Cell count and differential (5-10 mL, EDTA).

<u>**Syringe**</u> - pH (2 mL collected anaerobically, heparinized on ice)

<u>**Bag or Bottle**</u> - Cytology.

10. Other Orders and Meds:

HEMATOLOGY

ANTICOAGULANT OVERDOSE

Heparin Overdose:
1. Discontinue heparin infusion
2. Protamine sulfate, 1 mg IV for every 100 units of heparin infused in preceding 2h, dilute in 25-50 mL fluid IV over 10-20 min (max 50 mg in 10 min period). Watch for signs of anaphylaxis, especially if patient has been on NPH insulin therapy.

Warfarin (Coumadin) Overdose:
-Gastric lavage & activated charcoal if recent oral ingestion. Discontinue Coumadin and heparin and monitor hematocrit.

Minor Bleeds:
-Vitamin K (Phytonadione), 5-10 mg PO or 2.5-5 mg SQ or 10 mg IV doses q12h, titrated to desired INR check INR q12h until stable.

Serious Bleeds:
-Vitamin K (Phytonadione), 10-20 mg in 50-100 mL fluid IV over 30-60 min (INR q6h until stable) **OR**
-Fresh frozen plasma, 2-3 units (severe bleeds).

Labs: CBC, check platelets (if <50,000, transfuse 4-6 U platelets), PTT, INR.
Other orders and meds:

DEEP VEIN THROMBOSIS

1. **Admit to:**
2. **Diagnosis:** Deep vein thrombosis
3. **Condition:**
4. **Vital signs:** q shift; Call physician if BP systolic >160, <90 diastolic. >90, <60; P >120, <50; R>25, <10; T >38.5°C.
5. **Activity:** Bed rest with legs elevated.
6. **Nursing:** Guaiac stools, warm packs to leg prn; keep leg elevated; measure calf circumference qd; no intramuscular injections or aspirin products.
7. **Diet:** Regular
8. **IV Fluids:** D5W at TKO
9. **Special Medications:**

Anticoagulation:
-Heparin IV bolus 5000-10,000 Units (100 U/kg) IVP, then 1000-1500 U/h IV infusion (20 U/kg/h; 15 U/kg/h if ≥ 80) [25,000 U in 500 ml D5W (50 U/ml)]. Check PTT 6 hours after initial bolus; adjust q6h until PTT 1.5-2 times control (50-70 sec). Discontinue heparin when INR in therapeutic range for two consecutive days.

-Warfarin (Coumadin) 5-10 mg PO qd x 2-3 d, then titrate based on rate of rise of INR; maintain INR 2.0-3.0 (INR 3.0-4.5 if recurrent thrombosis). May initiate Coumadin on second day of heparin if the PTT is in therapeutic range; discontinue heparin when INR is therapeutic for two consecutive days.

10. Symptomatic Medications:
   -Propoxyphene/acetaminophen (Darvocet N100) 1-2 tab PO q3-4h prn pain
   -Docusate sodium (Colace) 100-200 mg PO qhs.
   -Ranitidine (Zantac) 150 mg PO bid.

11. Extras: CXR PA & LAT, ECG; impedance plethysmography & Doppler scan of legs, venography. V/Q scan.

12. Labs: CBC & INR/PTT, SMA 7. UA with dipstick for blood. PTT 6h after bolus & q4-6h until PTT 1.5-2.0 x control then qd. INR at initiation of warfarin & qd.

13. Other Orders and Meds:

PULMONARY EMBOLISM

1. Admit to:
2. Diagnosis: Pulmonary embolism
3. Condition:
4. Vital signs: q1h x 12h, then qid; Call physician if BP >160/90, <90/60; P >120, <50; R >30, <10; T >38.5°C; O2 sat < 90%
5. Activity: Bedrest with bedside commode
6. Nursing: Pulse oximeter, guaiac stools, O2 at 2-4 L by NC. No intramuscular injections; bed board, antiembolism stockings
7. Diet: Regular
8. IV Fluids: D5W at TKO.
9. Special Medications:
Anticoagulation:
   -Heparin IV bolus 5000-10,000 Units (100 U/kg) IVP, then 1000-1500 U/h IV infusion (20 U/kg/h; 15 U/kg/h if ≥ 80) [25,000 U in 500 ml D5W (50 U/ml)]. Check PTT 6 hours after initial bolus; adjust q6h until PTT 1.5-2 times control (60-80 sec). Discontinue heparin when INR in therapeutic range for two consecutive days.
   -Warfarin (Coumadin) 5 -10 mg PO qd x 2-3 d, then 2-5 mg PO qd based on rate of rise of INR. Maintain INR of 2.0-3.0 (INR 3.0-4.5 if recurrent pulmonary embolism). Check INR at initiation of warfarin & qd. May initiate Coumadin on second day of heparin if the PTT is in therapeutic range; discontinue heparin when INR is therapeutic for two consecutive days.

Thrombolytics (symptoms <48 hours, positive angiogram, no contraindications. Indicated if hemodynamically compromised):

> **Baseline Labs:** CBC, PT/PTT, fibrinogen.
>
> **Alteplase (Recombinant Tissue Plasminogen Activator, Activase):** 100 mg IV infusion over 2 hours, followed by heparin infusion at 15 U/kg/h (no loading dose) to maintain PTT 1.5-2.5 x control.
>
> **OR**
>
> **Streptokinase:** Pretreat with methylprednisolone 250 mg IVP and diphenhydramine (Benadryl) 50 mg IVP. Then give streptokinase, 250,000 units IV over 30 min, then 100,000 units/h for 24-72 hours. Initiate heparin infusion at 10 U/kg/hour (no loading dose); maintain PTT 1.5-2.5 x control.

10. Symptomatic Medications:
  -Meperidine (Demerol) 25-100 mg IV prn pain.
  -Docusate sodium (Colace) 100-200 mg PO qhs.
  -Ranitidine (Zantac) 150 mg PO bid.

11. Extras: CXR PA & LAT, ECG, VQ scan; pulmonary angiography; impedance plethysmography of lower extremities, Doppler scan of lower extremities.

12. Labs: CBC, INR/PTT, fibrinogen, SMA7, ABG, cardiac enzymes. UA with urine dipstick for blood. PTT 6 hours after bolus & q4-6h until PTT 1.5-2.5 x control, then. INR at initiation of warfarin & qd.

13. Other Orders and Meds:

SICKLE CELL CRISIS

1. **Admit to:**
2. **Diagnosis:** Sickle Cell Crisis
3. **Condition:**
4. **Vital signs:** q shift.
5. **Activity:** Bedrest
6. **Nursing:**
7. **Diet:** Regular diet, push oral fluids.
8. **IV Fluids:** D5½NS at 100-175 mL/h.
9. **Special Medications:**
  -Oxygen 2-4 L/min by NC or 30-100% by mask.
  -Meperidine (Demerol) 50-150 mg IM/IV/SC q4-6h.
  -Hydroxyzine (Vistaril) 25-100 mg IM/IV/PO q3-4h prn pain.
  -Morphine sulfate 10 mg IV/IM/SC q2-4h prn **OR** follow bolus by infusion of 0.05-0.1 mg/kg/h or 10-30 mg PO q4h **OR**
  -Acetaminophen/codeine (Tylenol 3) 1-2 tabs PO q4-6h prn.
  -Folic acid 1 mg PO qd.
  -Penicillin V (prophylaxis), 250 mg PO bid [tabs 125,250,500 mg].

Vaccination (especially if splenectomized):
-Pneumovax (23V) before discharge 0.5 cc IM x 1 dose; once in a lifetime.
-Influenza vaccine (Fluogen) 0.5 cc IM once a year.
10. Extras: CXR.
11. Labs: CBC, SMA 7, blood C&S, reticulocyte count, type & hold, parvovirus titers. UA, urine C&S.
12. Other Orders and Meds:

INFECTIOUS DISEASES

EMPIRIC THERAPY OF MENINGITIS

1. **Admit to:**
2. **Diagnosis:** Meningitis.
3. **Condition:**
4. **Vital signs:** q1-6h; Call physician if BP systolic >160/90, <90/60; P >120, <50; R>25, <10; T >39°C or less than 36°C
5. **Activity:** Bed rest with bedside commode.
6. **Nursing:** Respiratory isolation. I&O, daily weights, lumbar puncture tray at bedside.
7. **Diet:**
8. **IV Fluids:** D5W at TKO
9. **Special Medications:**

Meningitis Empiric Therapy 15-50 years old

-Ampicillin 2 gm IV q4h (with 3rd gen cephalosporin) **AND EITHER**
Ceftriaxone (Rocephin) 2 gm IV q12h (max 4 gm/d) **OR**
Cefotaxime (Claforan) 2 gm IV q4h **OR**
Ceftizoxime (Cefizox) 2 gm IV q4h **OR**
Ceftazidime (Fortaz) 2 gm IV q4h
-IV antibiotics x 10-14 days except in Listeria. Consider dexamethasone IV.

Empiric Therapy >50 years old, Alcoholic, Corticosteroids or Hematologic malignancy or other Debilitating Condition:

-Ampicillin 2 gm IV q4h **AND EITHER**
Cefotaxime (Claforan) 2 gm IV q4h **OR**
Ceftriaxone (Rocephin) 2 gm IV q12h (max 4 g/d) **OR**
Ceftizoxime (Cefizox) 2 gm IV q4h **OR**
Ceftazidime (Fortaz) 2 gm IV q4h
-Consider dexamethasone IV.

10. **Symptomatic Meds:**
-Acetaminophen 325-650 mg PO/PR q4-6h prn temp >101.
11. **Extras:** CXR, ECG, PPD with controls.
12. **Labs:** CBC, SMA 7 & 12, osmolality. Blood C&S x 2. UA with micro, urine C&S. Stool, throat, nasal C&S. Antibiotic levels peak & trough after 3rd dose.

    CSF Tube 1 - Gram stain of fluid (or of sediment if fluid is clear), C&S for bacteria (1-4 mL).

    CSF Tube 2 - Glucose, protein (1-2 mL).

    CSF Tube 3 - Cell count & differential (1-2 mL).

    CSF Tube 4 - Latex agglutination or counterimmunoelectrophoresis antigen tests for S. pneumoniae, H. influenzae (type B), N. meningitides, E. coli, group B strep, viral cultures, VDRL. India ink, fungal cultures, cryptococcal antigen, AFB (8-10 mL).

13. Other Orders and Meds:

_____

INFECTIVE ENDOCARDITIS

1. **Admit to:**
2. **Diagnosis:** Infective endocarditis
3. **Condition:**
4. **Vital signs:** q4h; Call physician if BP systolic >160/90, <90/60; P >120, <50; R>25, <10; T >38.5°C
5. **Activity:** Up ad lib
6. **Diet:** Regular
7. **IV Fluids:** Hep-lock with flush q shift.
8. **Special Medications:**

Subacute Bacterial Endocarditis Empiric Therapy:
   -Penicillin G 2-3 million U IV q4h or ampicillin 2 gm IV q4h **AND**
   Gentamicin 80 mg (1-1.5/mg/kg) IV q8h

Acute Bacterial Endocarditis Empiric Therapy
(including IV drug abuser):
   -Gentamicin 100-120 mg IV (2 mg/kg); then 80 mg (1-1.5 mg/kg) IV q8h **AND**
      EITHER
   Nafcillin or Oxacillin 2 gm IV q4h **OR**
   Vancomycin 500 mg IV q6h or 1 gm IV q12h (1 gm in 250 mL D5W over 1h q12h).

Streptococci viridans/bovis:
   -Penicillin G 2-3 million U IV q4h for 4 weeks **OR**
   -Vancomycin 1 gm IV q12h x 4 weeks **AND**
   Gentamicin 70 mg (1 mg/kg) q8h for first 2 weeks.

Enterococcus:
   -Gentamicin 70 mg (1 mg/kg) IV q8h x 4-6 weeks **AND**
   Ampicillin 2 gm IV q4h x 4-6 weeks.

Staphylococcus aureus (methicillin sensitive, native valve):
   -Nafcillin or Oxacillin 2 gm IV q4h x 4-6 weeks **OR**
   Vancomycin 1 gm IV q12h x 4-6 weeks **AND**
   Gentamicin 70 mg (1 mg/kg) IV q8h for first 3-5 days.

Methicillin resistant Staphylococcus aureus (native valve):
   -Vancomycin 500 mg IV q6h or 1 gm IV q12h (1 gm in 250 mL D5W over 1h q12h) x 4-6 weeks.

Staphylococcus epidermidis (native valve):
   -Vancomycin 500 mg IV q6h or 1 gm q12h x 4-6 weeks **AND**
   Gentamicin 70 mg (1 mg/kg) q8h for first 3-5 days **AND**
   Rifampin 600 mg PO qd x 6 weeks.

Methicillin sensitive Staph aureus (prosthetic valve):
   -Nafcillin or oxacillin 2 gm IV q4h x 6 weeks **AND**
   Rifampin 600 mg PO qd x 6 weeks **AND**
   Gentamicin 1 mg/kg IV q8h x 2 weeks.
Methicillin resistant Staph aureus (prosthetic valve):
   -Vancomycin 500 mg IV q6h or 1 gm IV q12h x 6 weeks **AND**
   Rifampin 600 mg PO qd x 6 weeks **AND**
   Gentamicin 1 mg/kg IV q8h x 2 weeks.
Staph epidermidis (prosthetic valve):
   -Vancomycin 500 mg IV q6h or 1 gm IV q12h x 6 weeks **AND**
   Rifampin 600 mg PO qd x 6 weeks **AND**
   Gentamicin 1 mg/kg IV q8h x 2 weeks.
Culture Negative Endocarditis:
   -Penicillin G 2-3 million U IV q4h x 4-6 weeks **OR**
   -Ampicillin 2 gm IV q4h x 4-6 weeks **AND**
   Gentamicin 80 mg (1-1.5 mg/kg) q8h x 2 weeks (or use nafcillin and gen-
      tamicin if Staph aureus suspected in drug abuser or prosthetic valve).
Fungal Endocarditis:
   -Amphotericin B 0.5 mg/kg/d IV (after test dose) + flucytosine 150 mg/kg/d
      PO.
9. Extras: CXR PA & LAT, echocardiogram, ECG.
11. Labs: CBC with differential, SMA 7 & 12. Blood C&S x 3-4 over 24h (if
septic, draw over 1h before starting antibiotic), serum cidal titers, minimum
inhibitory concentration, minimum bactericidal concentration. Repeat C&S in
48h, then q week. Antibiotic levels peak & trough at 3rd dose. UA, urine C&S.
12. Other Orders and Meds:

EMPIRIC THERAPY OF PNEUMONIA

1. **Admit to:**
2. **Diagnosis:** Pneumonia
3. **Condition:**
4. **Vital signs:** q4-8h; Call physician if BP >160/90, <90/60; P >120, <50; R>25, <10; T >38.5°C or O2 saturation <90%.
5. **Activity:**
6. **Nursing:** Pulse oximeter, I&O, Nasotracheal suctioning prn, incentive spirometry.
7. **Diet:** Regular.
8. **IV Fluids:** IV D5½NS at 125 cc/hr or TKO.
9. **Special Medications:**
   -Oxygen by NC at 2-4 L/min or 24-50% Ventimask or 100% non-rebreather (reservoir).

Community Acquired Pneumonia 5-40 years old without underlying lung disease:
   -Cefuroxime 25 mg/kg IV q8h (children) or 0.75-1.5 gm IV q8h (adults) **OR**
   -Ampicillin/sulbactam (Unasyn) 1.5-3.0 gm IV q6h **OR**
   -Clarithromycin (Biaxin) 250-500 mg PO bid 7-10 days **OR**
   -Azithromycin (Zithromax) 500 mg PO x 1, then 250 mg PO qd x 4 days **OR**
   -Erythromycin (Eramycin) 500 mg IV qid.

Community Acquired Pneumonia >40 years old:
   -Erythromycin 500 mg IV q6h **AND/OR**
   -Cefuroxime (Zinacef) 1.5 gm IV q8h **OR**
   -Cefotaxime (Claforan) 1-2 gm IV q8 **OR**
   -Ceftriaxone (Rocephin) 1-2 gm IV q12h **OR**
   -Trimethoprim/Sulfamethoxazole (Septra DS) 6-10 mg TMP/kg/d IV in 2-3 divided doses **OR**
   -Ampicillin/Sulbactam (Unasyn) 1.5 gm IV q6h.

COPD with pneumonia:
   -Erythromycin 500 mg IV q6h **AND**
   -Cefuroxime axetil (Ceftin) 250-500 mg PO bid **OR**
   -Cefotaxime (Claforan) 1-2 gm IV q4-6h **OR**
   -Ceftriaxone (Rocephin) 1-2 gm IV q12h **OR**
   -Ceftizoxime (Cefizox) 1-2 gm IV q8-12h **OR**
   -Cefuroxime (Zinacef) 0.75-1.5 gm IV q8h **OR**
   -Ampicillin/sulbactam (Unasyn) 1.5-3 gm IV q6h **OR**
   -Amoxicillin/clavulanate (Augmentin) 250-500 mg PO q8h **OR**
   -Ticarcillin/clavulanate (Timentin) 3.1 gm IV q4-6h (200-300 mg/kg/d).

Alcoholics, Diabetics, Heart Failure, Debilitated or other Underlying Diseases:
   -Erythromycin 0.5-1.0 gm IV q6h **AND EITHER**
   Cefotaxime (Claforan) 1-2 gm IV q4-6h **OR**

Ceftriaxone (Rocephin) 1-2 gm IV q12h **OR**
Cefuroxime (Zinacef) 0.75-1.5 gm IV q8h **OR**
Ceftizoxime (Cefizox) 1-2 gm IV q8 **OR**
TMP/SMX IV 6-10 mg TMP/kg per day in 2-3 divided doses **OR**
Ampicillin/Sulbactam (Unasyn) 1.5-3 gm IV q6h. **OR**
Ticarcillin/clavulanate Timentin 3.1 gm IV q4-6h (200-300 mg/kg/day).

Nosocomial, Hospital Acquired, Broad Spectrum Antibiotics Associated Pneumonia:

-Tobramycin 80-100 mg IV q8h (3-5 mg/kg/d) **AND EITHER**
Ceftriaxone 1-2 gm IV q12-24h **OR**
Ceftizoxime (Cefizox) or other 3rd generation cephalosporin (see above) **OR**
Piperacillin or Ticarcillin 3 gm IV q4-6h (with tobramycin or gentamicin) **OR**
Imipenem/cilastatin (Primaxin) 0.5-1.0 gm IV q6-8h.

Aspiration Pneumonia (community acquired):

-Clindamycin (Cleocin) 600-900 mg IV q8h (with or without gentamicin or 3rd gen cephalosporin) **OR**
-Ampicillin/Sulbactam (Unasyn) 1.5-3 gm IV q6h (with or without gentamicin or 3rd gen cephalosporin) **OR**
-Ticarcillin/Clavulanic acid (Timentin) 3.1 gm IV q4-6h (with or without gentamicin) **OR**
-Imipenem/Cilastatin (Primaxin) 0.5-1.0 gm IV q6-8h

Aspiration Pneumonia (nosocomial):

-Tobramycin 2 mg/kg IV then 1.7 mg/kg IV q8h **OR**
-Ceftazidime 1-2 gm IV q8h **AND EITHER**
Clindamycin (Cleocin) 600-900 mg IV q8h **OR**
Penicillin G 1-2 MU IV q4h **OR**
Ampicillin/Sulbactam or Ticarcillin/clavulanate, or Imipenem/cilastatin (see above).

10. Symptomatic Medications:
-Acetaminophen (Tylenol) 650 mg 2 tab PO q3-4h prn temp >101 or pain.
-Docusate sodium (Colace) 100-200 mg PO qhs.
-Ranitidine (Zantac) 150 mg PO bid.

11. Extras: CXR PA, LAT, ECG, PPD with control antigens (candida, mumps).

12. Labs: CBC with differential, SMA 7 & 12, ABG. Blood C&S x 2. Sputum gram stain, C&S. Methenamine silver sputum stain (PCP); AFB smear/culture; fungal prep (KOH). Aminoglycoside levels peak & trough at 3rd dose. UA, urine culture.

Cold agglutinins, titers for chlamydia pneumonia, mycoplasma, legionella

13. Other Orders and Meds:

SPECIFIC THERAPY OF PNEUMONIA

Pneumococcal pneumoniae Pneumonia:
- -Penicillin G 1-2 million units IV q4h **OR**
- -Erythromycin 500 mg IV q6h.

Staphylococcus aureus Pneumonia:
- -Oxacillin or Nafcillin 2 gm IV q4h **OR**
- -Vancomycin 500 mg IV q6h or 1 gm IV q12h (1 gm in 250 cc D5W over 1h q12h).

Klebsiella pneumoniae Pneumonia:
- -Gentamicin 1.5-2 mg/kg IV, then 1.0-1.5 mg/kg IV q8h (adjust for Azotemia).
  AND EITHER
  Ceftriaxone (Rocephin) 2 gm IV q12h **OR**
  Ceftizoxime (Cefizox) 1-2 gm IV q8h **OR**
  Ceftazidime (Fortaz) 1-2 gm IV q8h.

Haemophilus influenzae:
- -Ampicillin 1-2 gm IV q6h (beta-lactamase negative) **OR**
- -Cefuroxime 0.75-1.5 gm IV q8h (beta-lactamase pos) **OR**
- -Ceftizoxime (Cefizox) 1-2 gm IV q8h **OR**
- -Chloramphenicol 0.5-1.0 gm IV q6h.

Pseudomonas aeruginosa:
- -Tobramycin 1.5-2.0 mg/kg IV, then 1.5-2.0 mg/kg IV q8h (adjust for Azotemia) **AND EITHER**
  Piperacillin, Ticarcillin, Mezlocillin or Azlocillin 3 gm IV q4h **OR**
  Ceftazidime 1-2 gm IV q8h.

Mycoplasma pneumoniae:
- -Clarithromycin (Biaxin) 250-500 mg PO bid 7-10 days **OR**
- -Azithromycin (Zithromax) 500 mg PO x 1, then 250 mg PO qd x 4 days **OR**
- -Erythromycin 500 mg PO or IV q6h x 14-21 days.

Legionella pneumoniae:
- -Erythromycin 1.0 gm IV q6h x 21 days **AND**
  Rifampin 600 mg PO qd x 21 days.

Moraxella (Branhamella) catarrhalis:
- -Ampicillin/sulbactam (Unasyn) 1.5-3 gm IV q6h **OR**
- -Cefuroxime 0.75-1.5 gm IV q8h **OR**
- -Erythromycin 0.5-1.0 gm IV q6h x 21 days.

Anaerobic Pneumonia:
- -Penicillin G 1-2 MU IV q4h **OR**
- -Clindamycin (Cleocin) 600-900 mg IV q8h. **OR**
- -Metronidazole (Flagyl) 500 mg IV q6-8h.

13. Other Orders and Meds:

PNEUMOCYSTIS PNEUMONIA IN HIV INFECTED PATIENTS

1. **Admit to:**
2. **Diagnosis:** PCP pneumonia
3. **Condition:**
4. **Vital signs:** q2-6h; Call physician if BP >160/90, <90/60; P >120, <50; R>25, <10; T >38.5°C; 02 sat <90%
5. **Activity:**
6. **Nursing:** Pulse oximeter.
7. **Diet:** Regular, encourage fluids.
8. **IV Fluids:** D5½NS at 50-100 cc/h or TKO.
9. **Special Medications:**

PNEUMOCYSTIS CARINII PNEUMONIA:

-Trimethoprim/sulfamethoxazole (Bactrim, Septra) 15-20 mg/kg/day (based on TMP) PO or IV in 3-4 divided doses x 21 days; TMP-SMX is the drug of choice

-If moderately severe PCP (Pa02 <70 mm Hg): Give methylprednisolone 40 mg IV q8h or prednisone 40 mg PO bid for 5 days. Taper dose to one-half this amount for the next 5 days; then 20 mg qd for an additional 11 days, for a total of 21 days.

-Pentamidine (Pentam) 3-4 mg/kg IV qd x 21 days, with methylprednisolone as above. Pentamidine is an alternate treatment if inadequate response to TMP-SMX.

-Atovaquone (Mepron) 750 mg PO tid x 21 days. Use restricted to those with mild to moderate PCP who are refractory to or intolerant of TMP-SMX.

PCP prophylaxis (previous PCP or CD4 <200)

-TMP/SMX DS (160/800 mg) PO qd **OR**

-Pentamidine, 300 mg in 6 mL sterile water via Respirgard II nebulizer over 20-30 min q4 weeks; may pretreat with Albuterol 2.5 mg in 5 mL NS **OR**

-Dapsone (DDS) 50 mg PO qd, given 2-7 days per week, contraindicated in G-6-PD deficiency.

Antiretroviral Therapy:

-Zidovudine (Retrovir)(CD4 <500, symptomatic AIDS)100 mg PO q4 hours or 100 mg five times a day; some physicians prescribe 200 mg tid. Dosage may be reduced to 100 mg tid if side effects are intolerable, or if significant anemia [100-mg caps] **OR**

-Didanosine (DDI, Videx)200 mg PO bid for patients >60 kg; or 125 mg PO bid for patients <60 kg [100-mg, 150-mg buffered tablet may be mixed with water and taken on an empty stomach] **OR**

-Zalcitabine (DDC, Hivid) 0.375-0.75 mg PO q8h [0.375, 0.75 mg].

-**Post-exposure Prophylaxis**: Zidovudine, 200 mg PO q4h x 72h, then 200 mg 5 times/day x 25 days.

Zidovudine-Induced Neutropenia/Ganciclovir-Induced Leucopenia
  -Recombinant human granulocyte colony-stimulating factor (G-CSF, Filgrastim, Neupogen) 1-2 mcg/kg SQ qd until absolute neutrophil count 500-1000; indicated only if the patient's endogenous erythropoietin level is low.

10. Other Medications:
  -Ranitidine (Zantac) 150 mg PO bid.

11. Extras: CXR PA & LAT.

12. Labs: ABG, CBC, SMA 7 & 12. Blood C&S x 2. Sputum for Gram stain, C&S, AFB. Giemsa immunofluorescence for Pneumocystis, fungal C&S. Induce sputum with nebulized 3% saline after gargling with 3% saline.
CD4 count, VDRL, serum cryptococcal antigen, HBsAg, anti-HBs, toxoplasmosis titer. UA.

Bronchoscopic Considerations: Consider bronchoscopy if sputum non-diagnostic or CXR is atypical for PCP or if patient not responding to empiric PCP therapy.

13. Other Orders and Meds:

OPPORTUNISTIC INFECTIONS IN HIV INFECTED PATIENTS

Oral Candidiasis:
  -Fluconazole (Diflucan) Acute: 100-200 mg po qd; higher dosages might be necessary. Maintenance: 100-200 mg po once weekly or 50-100 mg po qd **OR**
  -Ketoconazole (Nizoral), acute: 400 mg po qd 1-2 weeks or until resolved. Maintenance: 200 mg po qd-bid for 7 consecutive days per month or qd if necessary. **OR**
  -Clotrimazole (Mycelex) troches 10 mg dissolved slowly in mouth 5 times/d **OR**
  -Nystatin (Mycostatin) 100,000 U/mL, swish and swallow 5 mL po q 6 hr or one 500,000-unit tablet dissolved slowly in mouth q6h.

Candida Esophagitis:
  -Fluconazole 200-400 mg po qd x 14-21 days; higher dosages might be required **OR**
  -Ketoconazole 200 mg po bid.
  -Maintenance with fluconazole (100 mg po qd) or ketoconazole (200 mg PO qd) may be required at the lowest effective dose.

Primary or Recurrent Mucocutaneous HSV
  -Acyclovir (Zovirax), 200-400 mg po 5 times a day for 10 days, or 5 mg/kg IV q8h OR In cases of acyclovir resistance, foscarnet, 40 mg/kg IV q8h, via infusion pump only, for 21 days.
  -Prophylaxis: Acyclovir (Zovirax) 400 mg PO bid.

Herpes Simplex Encephalitis:
-Acyclovir 10 mg/kg IV q8h x 10-21 days.

Herpes Varicella Zoster
-Acyclovir 10 mg/kg IV over 60 min q8h for 7-14 days **OR** 800 mg PO 5 times/d x 7-10 days.

Cytomegalovirus infections:
-Ganciclovir (Cytovene) 5 mg/kg IV (dilute in 100 mLs D5W over 60 min) q12h x 14-21 days for retinitis, colitis, esophagitis (concurrent use with zidovudine may increase hematological toxicity)

Suppressive Treatment for CMV:
-Ganciclovir 5 mg/kg IV qd, or 6 mg/kg 5 times/wk.

Toxoplasmosis:
-Clindamycin 600-900 mg po or IV qid plus pyrimethamine 25-75 mg po qd-qOD plus leucovorin calcium (folinic acid) 10-25 mg po qd for 6-8 weeks for acute therapy; lifetime suppression with highest tolerated dosage.

Suppressive Treatment for Toxoplasmosis:
-Pyrimethamine 25-50 mg PO qd with or without sulfadiazine 0.5-1.0 Gm PO q6h; and folinic acid 5-10 mg PO qd. **OR**
-Pyrimethamine 50 mg PO qd; and clindamycin 300 mg PO q6h; and folinic acid 5-10 mg PO qd.

Cryptococcus Neoformans Meningitis:
-Amphotericin B 0.7-1.0 mg/kg/d IV; amphotericin total dosage not to exceed 2 g, with or without 5-flucytosine 100 mg/kg po qd in at divided doses for first 2-4 weeks or until clinically improved, followed by fluconazole 400 mg po qd or itraconazole 200 mg po bid 6-8 weeks
OR
-Fluconazole 400-800 mg po qd for 8-12 weeks

Suppressive Treatment for Cryptococcus:
-Fluconazole (Diflucan) 200 mg PO qd indefinitely.

Active Tuberculosis:
-Isoniazid (INH) 300 mg PO qd; and rifampin 600 mg PO qd; and pyrazinamide 15-25 mg/kg PO qd; and ethambutol 15-25 mg/kg PO qd; or streptomycin 15 mg/kg IM qd, or 20 mg/kg IM twice/wk.
-Pyridoxine (Vitamin B6) 50 mg PO qd concurrent with INH.
-All four drugs are continued for 2 months; isoniazid and rifampin (depending on susceptibility testing) are continued for a period of at least 9 months and at least 6 months after the last negative cultures.

Prophylaxis for Inactive Tuberculosis:
-Isoniazid 300 mg PO qd; and pyridoxine 50 mg PO qd x 12 months.

Disseminated Mycobacterium Avium Complex (MAC):
-Clarithromycin (Biaxin) 500-1000 mg PO bid; or Azithromycin (Zithromax) 500 mg PO qd; **AND EITHER**
Ethambutol 15-25 mg/kg PO qd, **OR**
Clofazimine (Lamprene) 100-200 mg PO qd, **OR**

Ciprofloxacin (Cipro) 750 mg PO bid or 400 mg IV bid.

Prophylaxis for MAC:

-Rifabutin (Mycobutin), 300 mg PO qd or 150 mg PO bid.

Disseminated Coccidioidomycosis:

-Amphotericin B 0.5-0.8 mg/kg IV qd, until total dose 2.0-2.5 gms. **OR**

-Fluconazole (Diflucan) 400-800 mg PO and/or IV qd.

Disseminated Histoplasmosis:

-Amphotericin B 0.5-0.8 mg/kg IV qd, until total dose 15 mg/kg. **OR**

-Itraconazole (Sporanox) 200 mg PO bid.

-AIDS associated diarrhea - see page 62

Suppressive Treatment for Histoplasmosis:

-Itraconazole (Sporanox) 200 mg PO bid **OR**

-Amphotericin B 0.5-0.8 mg/kg IV q/wk.

Other Orders and Meds:

SEPTIC ARTHRITIS

1. **Admit to:**
2. **Diagnosis:** Septic arthritis
3. **Condition:**
4. **Vital signs:** q shift
5. **Activity:** No weight bearing on infected joint. Up in chair as tolerated. Bedside commode with assistance.
6. **Nursing:** Warm compresses prn, keep joint immobilized. Assist with passive range of motion exercises of the affected joint bid; otherwise, keep knee in resting splint; encourage ROM exercise of other joints
7. **Diet:** Regular diet (offer high-residue foods and prunes if patient is constipated).
8. **IV Fluids:** D5W TKO
9. **Special Medications:**

Empiric Therapy for Adults without Gonorrhea contact:

-Nafcillin or Oxacillin 2 gm IV q4h **AND**

Gentamicin 100-120 mg (1.5-2 mg/kg) IV, then 80 mg IV q8h (3-5 mg/kg/d) **OR**

-Vancomycin 500 mg IV q6h or 1 gm q12h (1 gm in 250 cc D5W over 60 min q12h) and Gentamicin as above **OR**

-Ticarcillin/clavulanate (Timentin) 3.1 gms IV q4-6h **OR**

-Ampicillin/Sulbactam (Unasyn) 1.5-3.0 gm IV q6h **OR**

-Imipenem/cilastatin (Primaxin) 0.5-1.0 gm IV q6-8h.

Empiric Therapy for Adults with possible Gonorrhea:

-Ceftriaxone (Rocephin) 1-2 gm IV q12h (max 4 gm/d) **OR**

-Ciprofloxacin (Cipro) 400 mg IV q12h.

10. Symptomatic Medications:
-Acetaminophen & codeine (Tylenol 3) 1-2 PO q4-6h prn pain.
-Heparin 5000 U SQ bid.
11. Extras: X-ray views of joint (AP and lateral), CXR, ECG. Culture. PPD. Physical therapy consult for exercise program.
12. Labs: CBC, SMA 7&12, blood C&S x 2, VDRL. UA. Cultures of urethra, cervix, urine, throat, sputum, skin, rectum. Antibiotic levels.

<u>Synovial fluid:</u>
   <u>Tube 1</u> - Glucose, protein, lactate, pH.
   <u>Tube 2</u> - Gram stain, C&S, fungal, AFB.
   <u>Tube 3</u> - Cell count.
13. Other Orders and Meds:

SEPTIC SHOCK

1. **Admit to:**
2. **Diagnosis:** Sepsis
3. **Condition:**
4. **Vital signs:** q1h; Call physician if BP systolic >160/90, <90/60; P >120, <50; R>25, <10; T >38.5°C; urine output < 25 cc/hr for 4h 02 saturation <90%.
5. **Activity:** Bed rest.
6. **Nursing:** I&O, pulse oximeter. Foley catheter to closed drainage.
7. **Diet:** NPO
8. **IV Fluids:** 2 liters of normal saline over 2 hours, then D5½ NS at 125 cc/h
9. **Special Medications:**
-Oxygen at 2-5 L/min by NC or mask.

<u>Non-immunocompromised Adults, Antibiotics:</u> If pelvic or intra-abdominal infection, use ampicillin or vancomycin with gent/tobramycin, add clindamycin or metronidazole **OR** use cefoxitin & gent/tobramycin **OR** Unasyn & gent/tobramycin). May use 3rd generation cephalosporins in place of aminoglycosides if resistant gram-neg pathogens are not suspected.
-Ceftazidime (Fortaz) 1-2 g IV q8h **OR**
-Ceftizoxime (Cefizox) 1-2 gm IV q8h **OR**
-Cefotaxime (Claforan) 2 gm q4-6h **OR**
-Ceftriaxone (Rocephin) 1-2 gm IV q12h (max 4 gm/d). **OR**
-Cefoxitin (Mefoxin) 1-2 gms q6-8h **OR**
-Cefotetan (Cefotan) 1-2 Gms IV q12h **OR**
-Cefotetan (Cefotan) 1-2 Gms IV q12h **OR**
-Ampicillin 2 gm IV q4h **OR**
-Piperacillin, ticarcillin or mezlocillin 3 gms IV q4-6h **AND**
-Gentamicin or tobramycin 100-120 mg (1.5-2 mg/kg) IV, then 80 mg IV q8h (3-5 mg/kg/d) **AND**

-Clindamycin 600-900 IV q8h (15-30 mg/kg/d) **OR**

-Metronidazole 500 mg (7.5 gm/kg) IV q6h **OR**

-Ticarcillin/clavulanic acid (Timentin) 3.1 gm IV q4-6h (200-300 mg/kg/d) (with gent/tobramycin). **OR**

-Ampicillin/Sulbactam (Unasyn) 1.5-3.0 gm IV q6h (with gent/tobramycin) **OR**

-Imipenem/cilastatin (Primaxin) 0.5-1.0 gm IV q6-8h (with gent/tobramycin).

-Vancomycin 500 mg IV q6h or 1 gm IV q12h.

Nosocomial sepsis with IV catheter or IV drug abuse

-Vancomycin 500 mg IV q6h or 1 gm q12h (1 gm in 250 cc D5W over 60 min q12h); **AND**

Gentamicin or Tobramycin as above; **AND EITHER**

Ceftazidime or Ceftizoxime 1-2 gms IV q8h **OR**

Piperacillin, ticarcillin or mezlocillin 3 gm IV q4-6h.

Blood Pressure Support

-Dopamine 4-20 mcg/kg/min (200 mg in 250 cc D5W, 800 mcg/mL).

-Albumin 25 gm IV (100 mL of 25% sln) **OR**

-Hetastarch (Hespan) 500-1000 cc over 30-60 min (max 1500 cc/d).

-Dobutamine (tissue oxygenation support; use in addition to agents need for BP support) 5 mcg/kg/min, and titrate up to max 15 mcg/kg/min to get maximum increase in cardiac index and oxygen transport without decreasing mean arterial pressure; goal is to improve SVO_2.

CANDIDA SEPTICEMIA:

-Amphotericin B, 1 mg test dose (D5W 100 mLs 60 min), then 10-20 mg (D5W 250 mLs over 3-4h) the same day, then 0.4-0.5 mg/kg/day (D5W 250-500 mLs over 4-6h); total dose 0.5-1.0 gm. Acetaminophen, diphenhydramine prior to amphotericin, and meperidine (Demerol) 25-50 mg IV prn chills during Amphotericin B infusion.

10. Symptomatic Medications:

-Acetaminophen 650 mg PR/PO q4-6h prn temp >101.

-Ranitidine (Zantac) 50 mg IV q8h or 150 mg PO bid.

11. Extras: CXR, KUB, sinus films, ECG. Indium/Gallium scan, ultrasound, lumbar puncture. Cardiology, critical care consult.

12. Labs: CBC with differential, SMA 7 & 12, blood C&S x 3, T&C for 3-6 Units PRBC, INR/PTT, drugs levels peak & trough at 3rd dose. UA. Cultures of urine, sputum, wound, IV catheters, ascitic fluid, decubitus ulcers, pleural fluid.

13. Other Orders and Meds:

PERITONITIS

1. **Admit to:**
2. **Diagnosis:** Peritonitis
3. **Condition:**
4. **Vital signs:** q1-6h; Call physician if BP >160/90, <90/60; P >120, <50; R>25, <10; T >38.5°C.
5. **Activity:** Bed rest with legs elevated, bedside commode.
6. **Nursing:** Guaiac stools.
7. **Diet:** NPO
8. **IV Fluids:** D5½ NS at 125 cc/h
9. **Special Medications:**

Spontaneous Bacterial Peritonitis (nephrotic or cirrhotic):

Option 1:
-Ampicillin 1-2 gms IV q 4-6h; (vancomycin 500 mg IV q6h or 1 gm IV q12h if penicillin allergic) **AND EITHER**
Cefotaxime (Claforan) 1-2 gm IV q4-6h **OR**
Ceftizoxime (Cefizox) 1-2 gms IV q8h **OR**
Gentamicin or Tobramycin 1.5 mg/kg IV, then 1 mg/kg q8h (adjust for renal function).

Option 2:
-Ticarcillin/clavulanate (Timentin) 3.1 gms IV q6h.

Option 3:
-Imipenem/cilastatin (Primaxin) 0.5-1.0 gm IV q6h.

Secondary Bacterial Peritonitis:

Option 1:
-Cefoxitin (Mefoxin) 2 gm IV q6-8h **OR**
-Ampicillin 1-2 gm IV q4-6h **AND**
Gentamicin or tobramycin (aminoglycosides are not recommended in patients with cirrhosis) 100-120 mg (1.5 mg/kg); then 80 mg IV q8h (5 mg/kg/d)(if resistant, use amikacin) **AND**
Metronidazole 500 mg IV q6h (15-30 mg/kg/d)

Option 2:
-Ticarcillin/clavulanic acid (Timentin) 3.1 gm IV q4-6h (200-300 mg/kg/d) with aminoglycoside as above.

Option 3:
-Ampicillin/sulbactam (Unasyn) 1.5-3.0 gm IV q6h with aminoglycoside as above.

Option 4:
-Imipenem/cilastatin (Primaxin) 0.5-1.0 gm IV q6-8h.

Fungal:
-Amphotericin B (2 mg/L 1st 24 hours then 1.5 mg/L) **AND**
Flucytosine (100 mg/L 1st 3 days then 30 mg/L)

10. **Symptomatic Meds:**

-Ranitidine (Zantac) 50 mg IV q8h or 150 mg PO bid.
-Acetaminophen 325 mg PO/PR q4-6h prn temp >101.

11. Extras: Plain film, upright abdomen, lateral decubitus, CXR PA & LAT; stat surgery consult for secondary bacterial peritonitis; ECG, abdominal ultrasound. CT scan.

12. Labs: CBC with differential, SMA 7 & 12, amylase, lactate. INR/PTT, UA with micro, C&S; drugs levels peak & trough 3rd dose.

PARACENTESIS TUBE 1 - Cell count & differential (1-2 mL, EDTA purple top tube)

TUBE 2 - Gram stain of sediment; inject 10-20 mL into anaerobic & aerobic culture bottle; AFB, fungal C&S (3-4 mL).

TUBE 3 - Glucose, protein, albumin, LDH, triglycerides, specific gravity, bilirubin, amylase (2-3 mL, red top tube).

SYRINGE - pH, lactate (3 mL).

13. Other Orders and Meds:

DIVERTICULITIS

1. **Admit to:**
2. **Diagnosis:** Diverticulitis
3. **Condition:**
4. **Vital signs:** qid; Call physician if BP systolic >160/90, <90/60; P >120, <50; R>25, <10; T >38.5°C
5. **Activity:** Up ad lib in room.
6. **Nursing:** Daily weights, I&O. Guaiac all stools.
7. **Diet:** NPO. Advance to clear liquids in morning as tolerated.
8. **IV Fluids:** 0.5-2 L NS over 1-2 hr then, D5½NS at 125 cc/hr. NG tube at low intermittent suction (if obstructed).
9. **Special Medications:**

Regimen 1:

-Gentamicin or tobramycin 100-120 mg IV (1.5-2 mg/kg), then 80 mg IV tid (5 mg/kg/d) **AND EITHER**

Cefoxitin (Mefoxin) 2 gm IV q6-8h **OR**

Clindamycin (Cleocin) 600-900 mg IV q8h.

Regimen 2:

-Metronidazole 1 g (15 mg/kg) IV then 500 mg q6-8h (15-30 mg/kg/d) **AND**

Ciprofloxacin (Cipro) 250-500 mg PO bid or 200-300 mg IV q12h

Outpatient Regimen:

-Trimethoprim/SMX (Bactrim DS) 1 double strength tab PO bid (and clindamycin or metronidazole PO) **OR**

-Ciprofloxacin (Cipro) 250-500 mg PO bid.

10. Symptomatic Medications:
   -Ranitidine (Zantac) 50 mg IV q8h or 150 mg PO bid.
   -Meperidine 50-100 mg IM or IV q3-4h prn pain.
   -Zolpidem (Ambien) 5-10 mg qhs, use 5 mg for elderly

11. Extras: Acute abdomen series, CXR PA & LAT, ECG, CT scan of abdomen, ultrasound, surgery and GI consults.

12. Labs: CBC with differential, SMA 7 & 12, amylase, lipase, blood cultures x 2, drug levels peak & trough 3rd dose. UA, C&S. Dipstick urine for blood.

13. Other Orders and Meds:

LOWER URINARY TRACT INFECTION

1. Admit to:

2. Diagnosis: UTI

3. Condition:

4. Vital signs: tid; Call physician if BP <90/60; >160/90; R >30, <10; P >120, <50; T >38.5°C

5. Activity:

6. Nursing:

7. Diet: Regular

8. IV Fluids:

9. Special Medications:

Lower Urinary Tract Infection:
   -Treat for three to seven days.
   -Trimethoprim/SMX (Septra DS) one double strength tab PO bid x 3-10 d **OR**
   -Amoxicillin 500 mg PO q8h x 3-10 d **OR**
   -Amoxicillin/clavulanate (Augmentin) 250-500 mg tab PO bid-tid **OR**
   -Nitrofurantoin (Macrodantin) 100 mg PO q6h **OR**
   -Norfloxacin (Noroxin) 400 mg PO bid x 3-10 d **OR**
   -Ciprofloxacin (Cipro) 250 mg PO bid x 3-10 d or 200 mg IV q12h **OR**
   -Ofloxacin (Floxin) 200 mg PO bid **OR**
   -Lomefloxacin (Maxaquin) 400 mg PO qd **OR**
   -Cephalothin (Keflex) 500 mg PO q6h **OR**
   -Cefadroxil (Duricef) 500 mg PO bid **OR**
   -Cefixime (Suprax) 200 mg PO q12h or 400 mg PO qd **OR**
   -Cefazolin (Ancef) 1-2 gm IV q8h.

Complicated or Catheter Associated Urinary Tract Infection:
   -Ampicillin 1 gm IV q4-6h **AND EITHER**
   Cefazolin (Ancef) 1-2 gm IV q8h **OR**
   Ceftizoxime (Cefizox) 1 gm IV q8h. **OR**
   Ceftriaxone (Rocephin) 0.5-1 gm IV q12h **OR**
   Aztreonam (Azactam) 1-2 gm IV q6-8h **OR**

Gentamicin 100-120 mg IV (1.5-2 mg/kg); then 80 mg IV q8h (1.5/kg q8-12h) **OR**

-Ticarcillin/clavulanic acid (Timentin) 3.1 gm IV q4-6h

-Ciprofloxacin or Norfloxacin (see above).

Prophylaxis (≥ 3 episodes/yr):

-Trimethoprim/SMX ½ single strength tab PO qd (after eradication of infection).

CANDIDA CYSTITIS

-Fluconazole (Diflucan) 100 mg PO or IV x 1 dose, then 50 mg PO or IV qd for 5 days **OR**

-Amphotericin B continuous bladder irrigation, 50 mg/1000 mL sterile water (50 mcg/mL) via 3-way Foley catheter at 1 L/d for 5 days.

10. Symptomatic Medications:

-Phenazopyridine (Pyridium) 100 mg PO tid.

11. Extras: Renal ultrasound, IVP.

12. Labs: CBC, SMA 7. UA with micro, urine Gram stain, C&S.

13. Other Orders and Meds:

PYELONEPHRITIS

1. **Admit to:**

2. **Diagnosis:** Pyelonephritis

3. **Condition:**

4. **Vital signs:** tid; Call physician if BP <90/60; >160/90; R >30, <10; P >120, <50; T >38.5°C

5. **Activity:**

6. **Nursing:** I&O.

7. **Diet:** Regular

8. **IV Fluids:** D5½ NS at 100 cc/h.

9. **Special Medications:**

-Ampicillin 1 gm IV q4-6h (if allergic, use vancomycin 500 mg IV q6h or 1 gm IV q12h) **AND EITHER**

Gentamicin or tobramycin - loading dose of 100-120 mg IV (1.5-2 mg/kg); then 80 mg IV q8h (2-5 mg/kg/d) **OR**

Ceftizoxime (Cefizox) 1 gm IV q8h **OR**

Ceftazidime (Fortaz) 1 gm IV q8h.

-Ticarcillin/clavulanate (Timentin) 3.1 gm IV q6h

-Ciprofloxacin (Cipro) 250-500 mg PO bid or 200 mg IV q12h.

-Norfloxacin (Noroxin) 400 mg PO bid.

-Amoxicillin/clavulanate (Augmentin) 250 mg or 500 mg tab PO tid.

-Trimethoprim/SMX (TMP-SMX, Septra) 160/800 mg (1 DS tab) PO bid or IV (10 mLs in 100 mLs D5W over 2h) q12h.

10. Symptomatic Medications:
  -Phenazopyridine (Pyridium) 100-200 mg PO tid.
  -Meperidine (Demerol) 50-100 mg IM q4-6h prn pain.
11. Extras: Renal ultrasound, IVP, KUB.
12. Labs: CBC with differential, SMA 7. UA with micro, urine Gram stain, C&S; blood C&S x 2. Drug levels peak & trough at 3rd or 4th dose.
13. Other Orders and Meds:

OSTEOMYELITIS

1. Admit to:
2. Diagnosis: Osteomyelitis
3. Condition:
4. Vital signs: qid; call physician if BP <90/60; T >38.5°C
5. Activity:
6. Nursing: Keep involved extremity elevated. Encourage range of motion exercises of upper and lower extremities tid.
7. Diet: Regular, high fiber.
8. IV Fluids: Hep-lock with flush q shift.
9. Special Medications:

Adult Empiric Therapy (staph a, gram neg, strep):
  -Nafcillin or Oxacillin 2 gm IV q4h **OR**
  -Cefazolin (Ancef) 1-2 gm IV q8h **OR**
  -Vancomycin 500 mg q6h or 1 gm q12h (1 gm in 250 cc D5W over 1h q12h)
  -**Add** 3rd generation cephalosporin if gram negative bacilli on Gram stain. Treat for 4-6 weeks

Post Operative or Post Trauma (staph aureus, gram neg, Pseudomonas):
  -Vancomycin 500 mg IV q6h or 1 gm q12h **AND** Ceftazidime (Fortaz) 1-2 gm IV q8h.
  -Imipenem/cilastatin (Primaxin)**(single drug Tx)** 0.5-1.0 gm IV q6-8h.
  -Ticarcillin/clavulanic acid (Timentin)**(single drug Tx)** 3.1 gm IV q4-6h (200-300 mg/kg/d).
  -Ciprofloxacin (Cipro) 500 mg PO bid or 200-300 mg IV q12h **AND** Rifampin 600 mg PO qd.
  -Treat for 4-6 weeks.

Osteomyelitis with Decubitus Ulcer:
  -Cefoxitin (Mefoxin), see above.
  -Ciprofloxacin (Cipro) and clindamycin or metronidazole.
  -Imipenem/cilastatin (Primaxin), see above.
  -Nafcillin, gentamicin and clindamycin; see above.
  -Treat for 4-6 weeks.

10. Symptomatic Medications:
  -Meperidine 50-100 mg IM q3-4h prn pain.
  -Docusate sodium (Colace) 100-200 mg PO qhs.
  -Heparin 5000 U SQ bid.

11. Extras: Technetium/Gallium bone scans, multiple X-ray views, CT/MRI.

12. Labs: CBC with differential, SMA 7, blood C&S x 3, MIC, MBC, UA with micro, C&S. Needle biopsy of bone for C&S and fungi; antibiotic levels peak & trough at 3rd dose. Urine culture.

13. Other Orders and Meds:

TUBERCULOSIS
(Immunocompetent Patient)

1. Admit to:

2. Diagnosis: Active Pulmonary Tuberculosis

3. Condition:

4. Vital signs: q shift

5. Activity: Up ad lib in room.

6. Nursing: Respiratory isolation for 1-2 weeks after starting treatment.

7. Diet: Regular

8. Special Medications:
  -Isoniazid 300 mg PO qd (5 mg/kg/d, max 300 mg/d) for 6 months **AND**
  -Rifampin 600 mg PO qd (10 mg/kg/d, 600 mg/d max) for 6 months **AND**
  -Pyrazinamide 1.5-2.0 gm (15-30 mg/kg/d, max 2 gm) PO qd for 6 months
  -If resistance to INH is likely, add Ethambutol 1.5 gm (25 mg/kg/d, 2.5 gm/d max) PO qd
  -The most widely used regimen is isoniazid, rifampin, and pyrazinamide for 2 months, then isoniazid and rifampin for 4 months.

Prophylaxis
  -Isoniazid 300 mg PO qd (5 mg/kg/d) x 6 months (12 months if HIV positive).

9. Extras: CXR PA, LAT, ECG.

10. Labs: CBC with differential, SMA7 & 12, LFT's, HIV serology. First AM sputum for AFB x 3 samples. UA with micro, C&S.

11. Other Orders and Meds:

CELLULITIS

1. **Admit to:**
2. **Diagnosis:** Cellulitis
3. **Condition:**
4. **Vital signs:** tid; Call physician if BP <90/60; T >38.5°C
5. **Activity:** Up ad lib.
6. **Nursing:** Keep affected extremity elevated; warm compresses prn.
7. **Diet:** Regular, encourage fluids.
8. **IV Fluids:** Hep lock with flush q shift.
9. **Special Medications:**

Empiric Therapy Cellulitis
- Nafcillin or Oxacillin 1-2 gm IV q4-6h **OR**
- Cefazolin (Ancef) 1-2 gm IV q8h **OR**
- Vancomycin 500 mg IV q6h or 1 gm q12h (1 gm in 250 cc D5W over 1h q12h) **OR**
- Erythromycin 500 IV/PO q6h **OR**
- Dicloxacillin 250-500 mg PO qid (in mild disease or after improvement on IV therapy); may add penicillin VK to enhance coverage for streptococcus.

Immunosuppressed, Diabetic Patients, or Ulcerated Lesions:
- Use nafcillin or cefazolin + (gent or aztreonam + clindamycin or metronidazole if septic) **OR** Timentin **OR** Imipenem **OR** Cipro + clindamycin or metronidazole.
- Nafcillin or oxacillin 1-2 gm IV q4-6h.
- Cefazolin (Ancef) 1-2 gm IV q8h.
- Cefoxitin (Mefoxin) 1-2 gm IV q6-8h.
- **If Septic:** Add gentamicin 100-120 mg IV (1.5-3 mg/kg), then 80 mg IV q8h (3-5 mg/kg/d) **OR** Aztreonam (Azactam) 1-2 gm IV q6-8h **PLUS**
- Clindamycin (Cleocin) 600-900 mg IV q8h or 450 mg PO qid **OR**
- Metronidazole (Flagyl) 500 mg IV/PO q6h.
- Ticarcillin/clavulanic acid (Timentin) **(single drug Tx)** 3.1 gm IV q4-6h (200-300 mg/kg/d).
- Ampicillin/Sulbactam (Unasyn)**(single drug therapy)** 1.5-3.0 gm IV q6h.
- Imipenem/cilastatin (Primaxin)**(single drug therapy)** 0.5-1 mg IV q6-8h **OR**
- Ciprofloxacin (Cipro) 250-500 mg PO bid or 200-300 mg IV q12h **AND** Clindamycin 250-500 mg PO bid or 600-900 mg IV q8h (or metronidazole).

10. **Symptomatic Medications:**
- Silver sulfadiazine or ½ strength Dakin's sln wet to dry dressings tid. 1:1000 Betadine soaks qd.
- Acetaminophen/codeine (Tylenol #3) PO q4h prn pain.

11. **Extras:** Technetium/Gallium scans, Doppler analysis (ankle-brachial indices), impedance plethysmography.

12. **Labs:** CBC, SMA 7, blood C&S x 2. Leading edge aspirate, swab, drainage fluid for Gram stain, C&S; UA, antibiotic levels.

13. Other Orders and Meds:

_____

PELVIC INFLAMMATORY DISEASE

1. **Admit to:**
2. **Diagnosis:** Pelvic Inflammatory Disease
3. **Condition:**
4. **Vital signs:** q4h x 24h then qid; Call physician if BP >160/90, <90/60; P >120, <50; R>25, <10; T >38.5°C
5. **Activity:**
6. **Nursing:** I&O.
7. **Diet:** Regular
8. **IV Fluids:** D5½NS at 100 cc/hr.
9. **Special Medications:**
   -Cefoxitin (Mefoxin) 2 gm IV q6h **OR** Cefotetan (Cefotan) 1-2 gms IV q12h;
      AND Doxycycline (Vibramycin) 100 mg IV q12h (IV for 4 days & 48h after
      afebrile, then complete 10-14 days of Doxycycline 100 mg PO bid) **OR**
   -Clindamycin 900 mg IV q8h **AND** Gentamicin 100-120 mg (2 mg/kg), then
      100 mg (1.5 mg/kg) IV q8h, then complete 10-14 d of Clindamycin 450 mg
      PO qid or Doxycycline 100 mg PO bid
10. **Symptomatic Medications:**
    -Acetaminophen (Tylenol) 325 mg 1-2 tabs PO q4-6h prn pain or temp >101.
    -Meperidine (Demerol) 25-100 mg IM q4-6h prn pain.
    -Zolpidem (Ambien) 10 mg PO qhs.
11. **Labs:** CBC, SMA 7 & 12, ESR. GC & chlamydia culture. UA with micro, C&S, VDRL, HIV; blood cultures x 2. Pelvic ultrasound.
12. **Other Orders and Meds:**

_____

NEUTROPENIC FEVER, ONCOLOGIC EMERGENCY
(PMN's <1000)

1. **Admit to:**
2. **Diagnosis:** Neutropenic fever
3. **Condition:**
4. **Vital Signs:** q2-4h: call M.D. if BP <90/60; >160/90; R >30 <10; P 7/20 <50; T >38.5° <36.0°
5. **Activity:** Bedrest with bathroom privileges
6. **Nursing:** I/O; change IV catheter/change Foley catheter: Send catheter tips for culture and Gram stain; strict reverse isolation; no flowers or plants at bedside.

7. **Diet:** Neutropenic precautions: no raw vegetable matter.

8. **IV Fluids:** D5½NS with 20 mcg KCL/L at 30 cc/h.

9. **Special Medications:**
   -Ceftazidime 2 gm IV q8h **OR**
   -Piperacillin **OR** Mezlocillin 3-4 gm IV q4h **AND**
   Gentamicin **OR** Tobramycin 2 mg/kg loading dose followed by 1.5 mg/kg
     q8h **AND**
   -Vancomycin 500 mg IV q6h (if staphylococcus infection is suspected) **AND**
   -Clindamycin 900 mg IV q8h (if mucositis or periodontal infection present).
     CONSIDER
   -Amphotericin B 0.5-0.7 mg/kg IV qd (after test dose) if persistent fever after
     5-7 days on broad spectrum antibiotics, consider empiric treatment for
     candida sepsis.

10. **Symptomatic Meds:**
    -Meperidine (Demerol) 25-100 mg IM/IV q4-6h prn pain.
    -Diphenhydramine (Benadryl) 25-50 mg PO qhs prn insomnia.
    -Mild of magnesia 30 cc PO q12h prn constipation.

11. **Extras:**
    -If indwelling central catheter, consider discontinuing and send for Gram
      stain, C&S; biopsy cutaneous lesions; thoracentesis, paracentesis, lumbar
      puncture, infectious disease consult.

12. **Labs:** CBC with differential, SMA7/12, INR/PTT; UA with micro; C&S/Gram
     stain.
    Oral, skin, soft tissue lesions - Gram stain, C&S, fungal culture.
    Stool - C&S, ova & parasites x 3; Wright's stain; CXR; blood cultures
    (aerobic/anaérobic/fungal) x 3. C. difficile toxin assay (if diarrhea due to recent
    antibiotic use).

13. **Other Orders/Meds:**

GASTROENTEROLOGY

PEPTIC ULCER DISEASE

1. **Admit to:**
2. **Diagnosis:** Peptic ulcer disease.
3. **Condition:**
4. **Vital Signs:** qid, postural BP; Call physician if BP systolic >160, <90; diastolic. >90, <60; P >120, <50; T >38.5°C
5. **Activity:** Up ad lib
6. **Nursing:** Guaiac all stools.
7. **Diet:** NPO 48h, then regular, no caffeine.
8. **IV Fluids:** D5½NS with 20 mEq KCL at 125 cc/h. NG tube at low intermittent suction (if obstructed).
9. **Special Medications:**
   -Ranitidine (Zantac) 50 mg IV bolus, then continuous infusion at 6.25-12.5 mg/h (150-300 mg in 500 mL D5W at 21 mL/h over 24h) or 50 mg IV q8h, or 150 mg PO bid or 300 mg PO qhs.
   -Cimetidine (Tagamet) 300 mg IV bolus, then continuous infusion at 37.5-50 mg/h (900 mg in 500 mL D5W over 24h) or 300 mg IV q6-8h, or 400 mg PO bid or 800 mg PO qhs.
   -Famotidine (Pepcid) 20 mg IV q12h or 20 mg PO bid or 40 mg PO qhs.
   -Nizatidine (Axid) 300 mg PO qhs or 150 mg PO bid.

Suppression or Eradication of H pylori:
   Triple-drug Therapy:
      -Bismuth Subsalicylate (Pepto-Bismol) 2 tabs or 30 mLs PO qid **AND**
      -Metronidazole (Flagyl) 250 mg PO tid **AND**
      -Tetracycline 500 mg qid or amoxicillin 500 mg qid. Treat for 10 to 14 days.
   Alternative Regimen:
      -Omeprazole, 20 mg bid **AND** tetracycline or amoxicillin, 1 gm PO bid, for 14 days.

10. **Symptomatic Medications:**
    -Trimethobenzamide (Tigan) 100-250 mg PO or 100-200 mg IM/PR q6h prn nausea **OR**
    -Prochlorperazine (Compazine) 5-10 mg IM/IV/PO q4-6h, or 25 mg PR q4-6h prn nausea.
    -Meperidine (Demerol) 50-100 mg IM/IV q3-4h prn pain
11. **Extras:** Upright abdomen, KUB, CXR, ECG, endoscopy. GI consult. Surgery consult.
12. **Labs:** CBC, SMA 7 & 12, amylase, lipase, LDH. UA. Fasting serum gastrin qAM x 3 day (hypersecretory syndrome). Salicylate level.
13. **Other Orders and Meds:**

GASTROINTESTINAL BLEEDING

1. **Admit to:**
2. **Diagnosis:** Upper/lower GI bleed
3. **Condition:**
4. **Vital signs:** q30min; central venous pressure q1h; Call physician if BP >160/90, <90/60; P >120, <50; R>25, <10; T >38.5°C; urine output <15 mL/hr for 4h; CVP >15 cm H_2O.
5. **Activity:** Bed rest
6. **Nursing:** Place nasogastric tube, then lavage with 2 L of room temperature normal saline, then connect to low intermittent suction, repeat lavage q1h. Record volume & character of lavage. Remove NG tube when there is no evidence of continued bleeding. Foley to closed drainage; I&O. Record stool character.
7. **Diet:** NPO
8. **IV Fluids:** Two 16 gauge IV lines. 3 L NS over 1-4h; when available, transfuse 2-6 units PRBC run as fast as possible, then call physician for further orders.
9. **Special Medications:**
   -Oxygen 2 L by NC.
   -Ranitidine (Zantac) 50 mg IV bolus, then continuous infusion at 6.25-12.5 mg/h [150-300 mg in 500 mL D5W over 24h (21 cc/h)], or 50 mg IV q6-8h **OR**
   -Cimetidine (Tagamet) 300 mg IV bolus, then continuous infusion at 37.5-50 mg/h (900 mg in 500 cc D5W over 24h), or 300 mg IV q6-8h **OR**
   -Famotidine (Pepcid) 20 mg IV q12h.

Suspected Esophageal Variceal Bleeds:
   -Vasopressin (Pitressin) 20 U IV over 20-30 minutes, then 0.2-0.3 U/min [100 U in 250 mL of D5W (0.4 U/mL)], for 30 min, followed by increases of 0.2 U/min until bleeding stops or max of 0.9 U/min. If bleeding stops, taper over 24-48h **AND**
   -Nitropaste (with vasopressin) 1 inch q6h **OR** nitroglycerin IV at 10-30 mcg/min continuous infusion (50 mg in 250 mLs D5W).
   -Vitamin K (Phytonadione) 10 mg IV/SQ qd for 3 days (only if INR is elevated).
   -Fresh frozen plasma 2-4 U IV (for severe coagulopathies or after transfusion of 6 U PRBC).
10. **Extras:** Potable CXR, upright abdomen, ECG. Surgery & GI consults.

Upper GI Bleeds: Esophagogastroduodenoscopy with possible coagulation or sclerotherapy; Sengstaken-Blakemore or Minnesota tube for tamponade (usually requires intubation).

Lower GI Bleeds: Sigmoidoscopy/colonoscopy (after a GoLytely purge 6-8 L over 4-6h), technetium 99m RBC scan, angiography with possible embolization.
11. Labs: Repeat spun hematocrit q2h with CBC with platelets q12-24h. Repeat PT in 6 hours. SMA 7 & 12, ALT, AST, alkaline phosphatase, salicylate level, INR/PTT, type and cross for 3-6 U PRBC & 2-4 U FFP.
12. Other Orders and Meds:

CIRRHOTIC ASCITES & EDEMA

1. **Admit to:**
2. **Diagnosis:** Cirrhotic ascites & edema
3. **Condition:**
4. **Vital signs:** Vitals, neurochecks & urine output q4-6 hours; Call physician if BP >160/90, <90/60; P >120, <50; T >38.5°C; urine output < 25 cc/hr x 4h, or abnormal mental status. Observe for confusion, tremulousness, tachycardia, seizures (alcohol withdrawal including delirium tremens), and notify physician if withdrawal signs occur.
5. **Activity:** Bed rest with legs elevated.
6. **Nursing:** I&O, daily weights, measure abdominal girth qd, guaiac all stools. No sedatives unless withdrawal signs appear.
7. **Diet:** 2500 calories, 100 gm protein; 500 mg sodium restriction; fluid restriction to 1-1.5 L/d (if hyponatremia, Na <130).
8. **IV Fluids:** Hep-lock with flush q shift.
9. **Special Medications:**
   - Diurese to reduce weight by 0.5-1 kg/d (if edema) or 0.25 kg/d (if no edema).
   - Spironolactone (Aldactone) 25-50 mg PO qid or 200 mg PO qAM, increase by 100 mg/d to max of 400 mg/d.
   - Furosemide (Lasix)(ascites refractory to above) 40-120 mg PO or IV qd-bid. Add KCL 20-40 mEq PO qAM.
   - Metolazone (Zaroxolyn) 5-20 mg PO qd.
   - Captopril (resistant ascites) 12.5-25 mg PO q8h.
   - Cimetidine (Tagamet) 300 mg PO tid-qid.
   - Vitamin K 10 mg SQ qd x 3d.
   - Folic acid 1 mg PO qd.
   - Thiamine 100 mg PO qd.
   - Multivitamin PO qd.

   Paracentesis: remove up to 5 L ascites if peripheral edema, tense ascites, or decreased diaphragmatic excursion. If large volume paracentesis, give salt-poor albumin 12.5 gm with each liter of fluid removed (50 mL of 25% solution); infuse 25 mL before paracentesis and 25 mL 6h after.

o see Hepatic Encephalopathy, page 68.

10. Symptomatic Medications:
  -Docusate sodium (Colace) 100-200 mg PO qhs.
11. Extras: KUB, CXR, abdominal ultrasound, liver-spleen scan, GI consult.
12. Labs: Ammonia, CBC, SMA 7 & 12, LFT's, albumin, LDH, GGT, amylase, lipase, blood C&S, INR/PTT, blood alcohol. Urine creatinine, Na, K.
Ferritin, TIBC (hemochromatosis), ceruloplasmin, urine copper (Wilson's disease) HBsAg, hepatitis B core IgM, anti-hepatitis B core antigen, anti-HBsAg/IgG, anti HC, Hepatitis C virus antibody, alpha-1-antitrypsin.

Ascitic Fluid
Tube 1 - Protein, albumin, specific gravity, glucose, bilirubin, amylase, lipase, triglyceride, LDH (3-5 mL, red top tube).
Tube 2 - Cell count & differential (3-5 mL, purple top tube).
Tube 3 - C&S, Gram stain, AFB, fungal (5-20 mL); inject 20 mL into blood culture bottles at bedside.
Tube 4 - Cytology (>20 mL).
Syringe - pH (2 mL).
Concomitant serum albumin, LDH, total protein, glucose.
13. Other Orders and Meds:

VIRAL HEPATITIS

1. Admit to:
2. Diagnosis: Hepatitis
3. Condition:
4. Vital signs: qid; Call physician if BP <90/60; T >38.5°C
5. Activity:
6. Nursing: Stool isolation, guaiac all stools.
7. Diet: Clear liquid (if nausea), low fat (if diarrhea).
8. Special Medications:
  -Cimetidine (Tagamet) 300 mg PO tid-qid
  -Vitamin K 10 mg SQ qd x 3d.
  -Multivitamin PO qd.
9. Symptomatic Meds:
  -Meperidine (Demerol) 25-100 mg IM q4-6h prn pain.
  -Prochlorperazine (Compazine) 5-10 mg PO/IM q4-6h prn.
  -Hydroxyzine (Vistaril) 25 mg IM/PO q4-6h prn nausea or pruritus.
  -Diphenhydramine (Benadryl) 25-50 mg PO/IV q4-6h prn pruritus.
10. Extras: Liver/spleen scan, ultrasound, GI consult.
11. Labs: CBC, SMA 7 & 12, GGT, LDH, 5'-nucleotidase, amylase, lipase, INR/PTT; acetaminophen level, anti-HA IgM, HBsAg, hepatitis C virus antibody, HBcAg, HBeAg, hepatitis core antibody, anti-HBe, anti-HBs, HDV-RNA, anti-

delta (IgM/IgG); alpha 1 antitrypsin level. ANA. Ferritin, TIBC, ceruloplasmin; urine copper.

12. Other Orders and Meds:

CHOLECYSTITIS

1. **Admit to:**
2. **Diagnosis:** Cholecystitis
3. **Condition:**
4. **Vital signs:** q4h; call physician if BP >160/90, <90/60; P >120, <50; R>25, <10; T >38.5°C
5. **Activity:** Bed rest with bedside commode.
6. **Nursing:** Daily weights, I&O.
7. **Diet:** NPO
8. **IV Fluids:** 0.5-2 L LR over 1-2h then D5½NS with 20 mEq KCL/L at 125 cc/hr. Levin NG tube (10-18 F) at low constant suction.
9. **Special Medications:**
   -Metronidazole 1.0 gm (15 mg/kg) over 1h, then 500 mg (7.5 mg/kg) IV q6h
     AND EITHER
   Mezlocillin, Azlocillin or Piperacillin 3 gm IV q4-6h **OR**
   Cefoxitin (Mefoxin) 1-2 gm IV q6-8h **OR**
   Cefotetan (Cefotan) 1-2 gm IV q12h.
   -Imipenem Cilastatin 0.5-1.0 gm IV q6h (single drug treatment).
   -Ampicillin/Sulbactam (Unasyn)**(single drug Tx)** 1.5-3 gm IV q6h.
   -Ticarcillin/Clavulanate (Timentin) **(single drug Tx)** 3.1 g IV q4-6h. In seriously ill patient consider adding aminoglycoside.
10. **Symptomatic Medications:**
    -Meperidine 50-100 mg IM q4-6h and Hydroxyzine (Vistaril) 25-50 mg IM q4h prn pain.
11. **Extras:** Right upper abdomen ultrasound (after 8 hour fast), HIDA scan, CXR PA & LAT, KUB, ECG. Surgical consult.
12. **Labs:** CBC, SMA 7 & 12, GGT, amylase, lipase, INR/PTT, hepatitis panel, type & cross match for 2 units PRBC. UA.
13. **Other Orders and Meds:**

BACTERIAL CHOLANGITIS & BILIARY SEPSIS

1. **Admit to:**
2. **Diagnosis:** Bacterial cholangitis
3. **Condition:**
4. **Vital signs:** q1-6h; Call physician if BP systolic >160, <90; diastolic. >90, <60; P >120, <50; R>25, <10; T >38.5°C
5. **Activity:** Bed rest
6. **Nursing:** I&O
7. **Diet:** NPO
8. **IV Fluids:** 0.5-3 L LR over 1-3h, then D5½NS with 20 mEq KCL/L at 125 cc/h. NG tube at low constant suction. Foley to closed drainage.
9. **Special Medications:**
   -Mezlocillin, Azlocillin or Piperacillin 3 gm IV q4-6h **AND**
   Metronidazole (Flagyl) 500 mg (7.5 mg/kg) IV q6h.
   -Cefoxitin (Mefoxin) 1-2 gm IV q6-8h (with gentamicin).
   -Ticarcillin/clavulanate (Timentin) 3.1 g IV q4-6h.
   -Ampicillin 1-2 gm IV q4-6h. **AND**
   Gentamicin 100 mg (1.5-2 mg/kg), then 80 mg IV q8h (3-5 mg/kg/d) **AND**
   Metronidazole 500 mg (7.5 mg/kg) IV q6h .
10. **Symptomatic Medications:**
    -Meperidine (Demerol) 25-100 mg IM q4-6h prn pain.
11. **Extras:** CXR, ECG, RUQ & ultrasound, HIDA scan, acute abdomen series. GI consult.
12. **Labs:** CBC, SMA 7 & 12, GGT, amylase, lipase, blood C&S x 2. UA, INR/PTT.
13. **Other Orders and Meds:**

ACUTE PANCREATITIS

1. **Admit to:**
2. **Diagnosis:** Acute pancreatitis
3. **Condition:**
4. **Vital signs:** q1-4h, call physician if BP >160/90, <90/60; P >120, <50; <10; T >38.5°C; urine output < 25 cc/hr.
5. **Activity:** Bed rest with bedside commode.
6. **Nursing:** Daily weights, I&O, fingerstick glucose qid, guaiac st
7. **Diet:** NPO
8. **IV Fluids:** 1-4 L NS over 1-3h, then D5½NS with 20 mEq KC
   NG tube at low constant suction (if obstruction). Foley to c

9. **Special Medications:**
   -Ranitidine (Zantac) 6.25-12.5 mg/h (0.2-0.4 mg/kg/h)(150- 300 mg in 500 mL D5W at 21 mL/h) IV or 50 mg IV q6-8h.
   -Cimetidine (Tagamet) 37.5-100 mg/h IV or 300 mg IV q6-8h.
   -Famotidine (Pepcid) 20 mg IV q12h.
   -Cefoxitin (Mefoxin) 1-2 gm IV q6-8h; antibiotics not required in uncomplicated pancreatitis.
   -Heparin 5000 U SQ q12h.
   -Total Parenteral Nutrition, if malnutrition or if NPO for >3-5 days; see page 66.

10. **Symptomatic Medications:**
    -Meperidine 50-100 mg IM q3-4h prn pain.

11. **Extras:** Upright abdomen, portable CXR, ECG, ultrasound, CT with contrast. Surgery and GI consults.

12. **Labs:** CBC, platelets, SMA 7 & 12, ionized & total calcium, triglycerides, amylase, lipase, LDH, AST, ALT, GGT; blood C&S x 2, HBsAg, INR/PTT, type & hold 4-6 U PRBC & 2-4 U FFP. Pancreatic isoamylase, immunoreactive trypsin, chymotrypsin, elastase, CA 19-9 antigen. UA, urine culture.

13. **Other Orders and Meds:**

EMPIRIC THERAPY OF DIARRHEA

1. **Admit to:**
2. **Diagnosis:** Diarrhea
3. **Condition:**
4. **Vital signs:** tid; call physician if BP >160/90, <80/60; P >120; R>25; T >38.5°C
5. **Activity:** Up ad lib
6. **Nursing:** Daily weights, I&O, stool volumes
7. **Diet:** NPO except ice chips x 24h, then low residual elemental diet; no milk products.

'V **Fluids:** 1-3 L NS over 1-3 hours; then D5½NS with 40 mEq KCL/L at 150 /h.

cial **Medications:**

r gross blood in stool or neutrophils on microscopic exam or

cin (Cipro) 500 mg PO bid x 10-14 days **OR**

(Noroxin) 400 mg PO bid **OR**

xin) 300 mg bid **OR**

mg qd for 3-5 days **OR**

X (Bactrim DS) one double strength (160/800 mg) tab PO

Symptomatic Meds if indicated:
- Kaopectate 60-90 cc PO qid or after each loose BM prn **OR**
- Loperamide (Imodium) 2-4 mg PO tid-qid prn, max 16 mg/d **OR**
- Diphenoxylate HCL (Lomotil) 1-2 tabs PO qid, max 12 tabs/day.
- Pepto Bismol 30 cc PO q30min x 8 hours.

11. Extras: Upright abdomen. GI consult.

12. Labs: SMA7 & 12, CBC with differential, UA, blood culture x 2. Amebic serum titers, HIV test.

Stool studies: Wright's stain for fecal leukocytes, ova & parasites x 3, C difficile toxin & culture, C&S, E coli 0157:H7 culture.

13. Other Orders & Meds:

SPECIFIC THERAPY OF DIARRHEA

Shigella:
- Trimethoprim/SMX, (Bactrim) double strength tab PO bid x 3-5 days.

Salmonella (bacteremia):
- Ofloxacin (Oflox) 400 mg IV/PO q12h x 14 days **OR**
- Ciprofloxacin (Cipro) 400 mg IV q12h or 750 mg PO q12h x 14 days **OR**
- Trimethoprim/SMX (Bactrim) DS tab PO bid x 14 days **OR**
- Ceftriaxone (Rocephin) 2 gms IV q12h x 14 days.

Campylobacter jejuni:
- Erythromycin 250 mg PO qid x 5-10 days

Enterotoxic/Enteroinvasive E coli (Travelers Diarrhea):
- Ciprofloxacin 500 mg PO bid x 5-7 days **OR**
- Trimethoprim/SMX (Bactrim), double strength tab PO bid x 5-7 days.

ANTIBIOTIC ASSOCIATED & PSEUDOMEMBRANOUS COLITIS; (Clostridium difficile)(discontinue offending antibiotic):
- Metronidazole (Flagyl) 250 mg PO or IV qid x 10-14 days **OR**
- Vancomycin 125 mg PO qid x 10 days (500 PO qid x 10-14 days, if recurrent).

AIDS ASSOCIATED DIARRHEA (severe refractory secretory diarrhea):
- Octreotide (Sandostatin) 200-300 mcg SQ in 2-4 divided doses x 2 weeks.

Yersinia Enterocolitica (sepsis):
- Trimethoprim/SMX (Bactrim), double strength tab PO bid x 5-7 days **OR**
- Ciprofloxacin 500 mg PO bid x 5-7 days **OR**.
- Ofloxacin (Floxin) 400 mg PO bid.

Entamoeba Histolytica (Amebiasis):

Mild to Moderate Intestinal Disease:
- Metronidazole (Flagyl) 750 mg PO tid x 10 days **OR**
- Tinidazole 2 gm per day PO x 3 days. **Followed By:**
- Iodoquinol 650 mg PO tid x 20 days **OR**

-Paromomycin 25-30 mg/kg/d PO in 3 divided doses x 7 days.

Severe Intestinal Disease:

-Metronidazole 750 mg PO tid x 10 days **OR**

-Tinidazole 600 mg PO bid x 5 days **Followed By:**

-Iodoquinol 650 mg PO tid x 20 days **OR**

-Paromomycin 25-30 mg/kg/d PO in 3 divided doses x 7 days.

Giardia Lamblia:

-Quinacrine HCL 100 mg PO tid x 5d **OR**

-Metronidazole 250 mg PO tid x 7 days.

Isospora Belli:

-Trimethoprim/SMX (Bactrim), 4 single strength tabs PO bid x 2-3 weeks.

Cryptosporidium:

-Paromomycin 500 mg po qid for 7-10 days [250 mg].

Other Orders & Meds:

CROHN'S DISEASE

1. **Admit to:**
2. **Diagnosis:** Crohn's disease.
3. **Condition:**
4. **Vital signs:** q4-6h; call physician if BP >160/90, <90/60; P >120, <50; R>25, <10; T >38.5°C
5. **Activity:** Up ad lib in room.
6. **Nursing:** Daily weights, I&O. NG at low intermittent suction (if obstruction).
7. **Diet:** NPO except for ice chips and medications x 48h, then low residue or elemental diet, no milk products.
8. **IV Fluids:** 1-3 L NS over 1-3h, then D5 ½ NS with 40 mEq KCL/L at 150 cc/hr.
9. **Special Medications:**

   -Prednisone 40-60 mg/d PO in divided doses **OR**

   -Hydrocortisone 50-100 mg IV q6h.

   -Sulfasalazine (Azulfidine) 0.5-1 gm PO bid; increase over 10 d to 0.5-1 gm PO qid **OR**

   -Olsalazine (Dipentum) 500 mg PO bid

   -Metronidazole 250-500 mg PO q6h.

   Other Medications:

   -B12, 100 mcg IM x 5d then 100-200 mcg IM q month.

   -Multivitamin PO qAM or 1 ampule IV qAM.

   -Folate 1 mg PO qd. (especially is sulfasalazine used)

10. **Extras:** Upright abdomen. CXR. colonoscopy. GI consult.
11. **Labs:** CBC, SMA 7 & 12, Mg, ionized calcium, liver panel, blood C&S x 2; ol Wright's stain.

12. Other Orders and Meds:

ULCERATIVE COLITIS

1. **Admit to:**
2. **Diagnosis:** Ulcerative colitis/Crohn's disease.
3. **Condition:**
4. **Vital signs:** q4-6h; call physician if BP >160/90, <90/60; P >120, <50; R>25, <10; T >38.5°C
5. **Activity:** Up ad lib in room.
6. **Nursing:** Daily weights, I&O. NG at low intermittent suction (if obstruction).
7. **Diet:** NPO except for ice chips x 48h, then low residue or elemental diet, no milk products.
8. **IV Fluids:** 1-3 L NS over 1-3h, then D5 ½ NS with 40 mEq KCL/L at 150 cc/hr.
9. **Special Medications:**
   -Sulfasalazine (Azulfidine) 0.5-1 gm PO bid, increase over 10 d as tolerated to 0.5-1.0 gm PO qid **OR**
   -Olsalazine (Dipentum) 500 mg PO bid **OR**
   -5-aminosalicylate (Mesalamine) 400-800 mg PO tid or 1 gm PO qid or enema 4 gm/60 mL PR qhs (retain for 8h)
   -Hydrocortisone retention enema, 100 mg in 120 mL saline bid
   -Methylprednisolone 10-20 mg IV q6h **OR**
   -Hydrocortisone 100 mg IV q6h **OR**
   -Prednisone 40-60 mg/d PO in divided doses.
   Other Medications:
   -B12, 100 mcg IM x 5d then 100-200 mcg IM q month.
   -Multivitamin PO qAM or 1 ampule IV qAM.
   -Folate 1 mg PO qd. (especially is sulfasalazine used)
10. **Symptomatic Medications:**
    -Loperamide (Imodium) 2-4 mg PO tid-qid prn, max 16 mg/d (not in acute phase) **OR**
    -Kaopectate 60-90 mL PO qid prn.
11. **Extras:** Upright abdomen. CXR. colonoscopy. GI consult.
12. **Labs:** CBC, SMA 7 & 12, Mg, ionized calcium, liver panel, blood C&S x 2; stool Wright's stain, stool for ova and parasites and enteric pathogens; urine culture; type and crossmatch for 2 units packed red blood cells.
13. **Other Orders and Meds:**

PARENTERAL NUTRITION

General Considerations: Daily weights, I&O. Finger stick glucose qid.
Peripheral Parenteral Supplementation:
  -3% amino acid sln (ProCalamine) up to 3 L/d at 125 cc/h **OR**
  -Combine 500 mL amino acid solution 7% or 10% (Aminosyn) & 500 mL 20%
    dextrose & electrolyte additive. Infuse at up to 100 cc/hr in parallel with:
  -Intralipid 10% or 20% at 1 mL/min for 15 min (test dose); if no adverse
    reactions, infuse 500 mL/d at 21 mLs/h over 24h, or up to 100 mLs/h over
    5 hours daily.
  -Draw triglyceride level 6h after end of Intralipid infusion.
Central Parenteral Nutrition:
  -Infuse 40-50 mL/h of amino acid-dextrose solution in the first 24h; increase
    daily by 40 mL/hr increments until providing 1.3-2 x basal energy require-
    ment & 1.2-1.7 gm protein/kg/d (see formula page 97).
Standard solution:

Amino acid sln (Aminosyn) 7-10%	500 mL
Dextrose 40-70%	500 mL
Sodium	35 mEq
Potassium	36 mEq
Chloride	35 mEq
Calcium	4.5 mEq
Phosphate	9 mMol
Magnesium	8.0 mEq
Acetate	82-104 mEq
Multi-Trace Element Formula	1 mL/d
(Zn, copper, manganese, chromium)	
Regular insulin (if indicated)	10-60 U/L
Multivitamin(12)(2 amp)	10 mL/d
(vitamin C, A, D, E, B12, thiamine, riboflavin, pyridoxine, niacinamide, pantothenate, biotin, folate)	
Vitamin K (in solution, SQ, IM)	10 mg/week
Vitamin B12	1000 mcg/week

WITH OR WITHOUT:
Intralipid 20% 500 mL/d IVPB; infuse in parallel with standard solution at 1
  mL/min x 15 min; if no adverse reactions, increase to 100 mL/hr. Obtain
  serum triglyceride 6h after end of infusion (maintain <250 mg/dL).
CYCLIC TPN 12h night schedule; Taper continuous infusion in morning by
  reducing rate to half original rate for 1 hour. Further reduce rate by half for an
  additional hour, then discontinue. Finger stick glucose q4-6h; Restart TPN
  afternoon. Taper at beginning & end of cycle. Final rate of 185 mL/hr for
  h and 2 hours of taper at each end for total of 2000 mL.
Special Medications:
  Cimetidine (Tagamet) 300 mg IV q6-8h or in TPN **OR**

-Ranitidine (Zantac) 50 mg IV q6-8h or in TPN bid.

-Insulin sliding scale.

8. Extras: Nutrition consult.

9. Labs:

    <u>Baseline</u> - draw all labs below.

    <u>Daily labs</u> - SMA7, osmolality, CBC, cholesterol, triglyceride (6 h after infusion), urine glucose & specific gravity.

    <u>Twice weekly Labs</u> - Cal, phosphate, SMA-12

    <u>Weekly Labs when indicated</u> - Protein, Mg, iron, TIBC, transferrin, INR/PTT, zinc, copper, B12, Folate, 24h urine nitrogen & creatinine. Prealbumin, retinol-binding protein.

10. Other Orders and Meds:

ENTERAL NUTRITION

General Considerations: Daily weights, I&O, nasoduodenal feeding tube. HOB at 30° while enteral feeding & 2 hours after completion. Record bowel movements.

<u>**Enteral Bolus Feeding**</u> - Give 50-100 mL of enteral solution (Jevity, Vionex, Osmolite) q3h initially. Increase amount in 50 mL steps to max of 250-300 mL q3-4h; 30 kcal of nonprotein calories/kg/d & 1.5 gm protein/kg/d. Before each feeding measure residual volume, and delay feeding by 1h if >100 mL. Flush tube with 100 cc of water after each bolus.

<u>**Continuous enteral infusion**</u> - Initial enteral solution (Jevity, Vionex, Osmolite) 30 mL/hr. Measure residual volume q1h x 12h then tid; hold feeding for 1h if >100 mL. Increase rate by 25-50 mL/hr at 24 hr intervals as tolerated until final rate of 50-100 mL/hr as tolerated. 3 Tablespoonfuls of protein powder (Promix) may be added to each 500 cc of solution. Flush tube with 100 cc water q8h.

Special Medications:

    -Metoclopramide (Reglan) 10-20 mg PO or in J tube q6h.

    -Cimetidine (Tagamet) 400 mg PO bid **OR**

    -Ranitidine (Zantac)150 mg PO bid.

Symptomatic Medications:

    -Loperamide (Imodium) 2-4 mg PO/J-tube q6h, max 16

    -Diphenoxylate/atropine (Lomotil) 1-2 tabs or 5-10 mL ⌐ tube q4-6h prn, max 12 tabs/d **OR**

    -Codeine sulfate 30 mg PO or in J-tube q6h.

    -Kaopectate 30 cc PO or in J-tube q8h.

Extras: CXR, plain film for tube placement, n⌐

Labs:
  Daily labs - SMA7, osmolality, CBC, cholesterol, triglyceride. SMA-12
  Weekly Labs when indicated - Protein, Mg, INR/PTT, 24h urine nitrogen &
    creatinine. Pre-albumin, retinol-binding protein.
Other Orders and Meds:

___

HEPATIC ENCEPHALOPATHY

1. **Admit to:**
2. **Diagnosis:** Hepatic encephalopathy
3. **Condition:**
4. **Vital signs:** q1-4h, neurochecks q4h; Call physician if BP >160/90,<90/60;
   P >120,<50; R>25,<10; T >38.5°C
5. **Allergies:** Avoid sedatives, diuretics, NSAIDS or hepatotoxic drugs.
6. **Activity:** Bed rest.
7. **Nursing:** Keep head-of-bed at 40 degrees, guaiac stools; turn patient q2h
   while awake, chart stools and notify physician if patient does not have a stool
   at least twice a day. Seizure precautions, egg crate mattress, soft restraints
   prn. Record inputs and outputs.
8. **Diet:** Nasogastric enteral feedings at 30 mL/hr. Increase rate by 25-50 mL/hr
   at 24 hr intervals as tolerated until final rate of 50-100 mL/hr as tolerated. No
   dietary protein for 8 hours. Give 2000 calories per day.
9. **IV Fluids:** D5W at TKO, Foley to closed drainage.
10. **Special Medications:**
   -Sorbitol 500 mL in 200 mL of water PO now.
   -Lactulose 30-45 mL PO q1h x 3 doses, then 15-45 mL PO bid-qid titrate to
     produce 3 soft stools/d **OR**
   ‗actulose enema 300 mL in 700 mL of tap water bid-qid, (may use rectal
     ‗‗oon catheter to retain 30-60 min, left side Trendelenburg x 15 min, then
       ‗‗ide with head elevated); may give cleansing Fleet enema x 2 before
          AND
           ‗gm PO q4-6h (4-12 g/d) **OR**
            (Flagyl) 250 mg PO q6h.
             ‗) 50 mg IV q6-8h or 150 mg PO bid **OR**
              ‗t) 300 mg IV q6-8h or 300 mg PO tid-qid **OR**
               ‗ mg IV/PO q12h.
                ‗ ampule IV qAM.

                  ‗f elevated PT (INR)
                   consults.

12. Labs: Ammonia, CBC, platelets, SMA 7 & 12, Mg, Cal, AST, ALT, GGT, LDH, alkaline phosphatase, protein, albumin, bilirubin, INR/PTT, ABG, blood C&S x 2, hepatitis panel. UA.

13. Other Orders and Meds:

ALCOHOL WITHDRAWAL

1. **Admit to:**
2. **Diagnosis:** Alcohol withdrawals / Delirium tremens.
3. **Condition:**
4. **Vital signs:** q4-6h; Call physician if BP >160/90, <90/60; P >130, <50; R>25, <10; T >38.5°C; or increase in agitation, confusion, tremor, or change in neurological status.
5. **Activity:**
6. **Nursing:** Seizure precautions. Soft restraints prn.
7. **Diet:** Regular, push fluids.
8. **IV Fluids:** Hep-lock or D5½NS at 100-175 cc/h.
9. **Special Medications:**
   <u>Withdrawal syndrome:</u>
   -Chlordiazepoxide (Librium) 50-100 mg PO/IV q6h x 3 days <u>OR</u>
   -Diazepam (Valium) 5-20 mg PO/IV q6-8h
   <u>Delirium tremens:</u>
   -Chlordiazepoxide 100 mg slow IV push or PO, repeat q4-6h prn agitation or tremor x 24h; max 500 mg/d. Then give 50-100 mg PO q6h prn agitation or tremor <u>OR</u>
   -Diazepam (Valium) 5 mg slow IV push repeat q6h until calm, then 5-10 mg PO q4-6h.
   <u>Seizures:</u>
   -Diazepam 5-10 mg IV q5-15 min prn seizures, may repeat 5 mg q10-15min prn; max dose 30 mg.
10. **Symptomatic Medications:**
    -Magnesium sulfate 1-8 gm in 100 mL D5W over 2-8h qd.
    -Multivitamin 1 amp IV, then 1 tab PO qd.
    -Folate 1 mg PO qd.
    -Thiamine 100 mg PO qd.
    -Acetaminophen 625 mg PO q4-6h prn headache.
    -Metoclopramide (Reglan) 10 mg PO/IV q6h prn nausea.
11. **Extras:** CXR, ECG. Alcohol rehabilitation & social work consult.
12. **Labs:** CBC, SMA 7 & 12, Mg, amylase, lipase, liver panel, VDRL, u drug screens. UA, INR/PTT.
13. **Other Orders and Meds:**

TOXICOLOGY

POISONING & DRUG OVERDOSE

DECONTAMINATION:
Ipecac (not if ingestion of acid/base, caustics, tricyclics, or if obtundent, impaired gag reflex, seizing):
-Ipecac syrup (only if <1h after ingestion), 30 mL with 240-480 mL liquid; may repeat x 1 after 30 minutes if no emesis.

Gastric Lavage: Place patient left side down, place nasogastric tube and check position by injecting air & auscultating. NS lavage until clear fluid, then leave activated charcoal or other antidote prn. Gastric lavage is contraindicated for corrosives.

Cathartics:
-Magnesium citrate 6% sln 150-300 mL PO
-Magnesium sulfate 10% solution 150-300 mL PO.

Activated Charcoal: 50 gm PO (first dose should be given using product containing sorbitol as cathartic). Repeat q2-6h if indicated.

Hemodialysis: Indicated for isopropanol, methanol, ethylene glycol, severe salicylate intoxication (>100 mg/dL), lithium, theophylline (if neurotoxicity, seizures, or coma).

ANTIDOTES:
NARCOTIC OR PROPOXYPHENE OVERDOSE:
-Naloxone hydrochloride (Narcan) 0.4 mg IV/ET/IM/SC, may repeat q2min.

METHANOL OR ETHYLENE GLYCOL OVERDOSE:
-Ethanol 60-80 mL (10% inj sln) IV over 30min, then 0.8-1.4 mL/kg/h. Maintain ethanol level 100-150 mg/100 mL.

CARBON MONOXIDE OVERDOSE:
-Hyperbaric oxygen therapy or 100% oxygen by mask if hyperbaric oxygen not available.

PHENOTHIAZINE OR EXTRAPYRAMIDAL REACTION:
-Diphenhydramine (Benadryl) 25-50 mg IV/IM q6h x 4 doses; followed by 25-50 mg IV/PO q6h for 24-72h prn **OR**
-Benztropine (Cogentin) 1-2 mg IV, then 1-2 mg IV/PO bid prn.

BENZODIAZEPINE OVERDOSE (Diazepam, midazolam, lorazepam, alprazolam):
-Flumazenil (Romazicon) 0.2 mg (2 mL) IV over 30 seconds q1min until a total dose of 3 mg; if a partial response occurs, continue 0.5 mg doses until a total of 5 mg. If the patient has continued sedation (respiratory depression does not reverse appreciably), repeat the above regimen or start a continuous IV infusion 0.1-0.5 mg/h. Excessive doses, beyond reversal of sedation, may cause seizures.

Drug screen (serum, gastric, urine); blood levels, SMA 7, fingerstick , CBC, LFT's, ECG.

Other Orders and Meds:

ACETAMINOPHEN OVERDOSE

1. **Admit to:** Medical intensive care unit.
2. **Diagnosis:** Acetaminophen overdose
3. **Condition:**
4. **Vital signs:** q1-4h with neurochecks; Call physician if BP >160/90, <90/60; P >130, <50 <50; R>25, <10; urine output <20 cc/h for 3 hours.
5. **Activity:** Bed rest with bedside commode.
6. **Nursing:** I&O, aspiration & seizure precautions. Place large bore (Ewald) NG tube, then lavage with 2 L of NS.
7. **Diet:** NPO
8. **IV Fluids:**
9. **Special Medications:**
   -Activated Charcoal 30-100 gm doses, remove via NG suction prior to acetylcysteine.
   -Acetylcysteine (Mucomyst, NAC) loading 140 mg/kg PO, then 70 mg/kg PO q4h x 17 doses (dilute to 5% sln)(follow acetaminophen levels) **OR** IV acetylcysteine 150 mg/kg in 200 mL D5W IV over 15 min, followed by 50 mg/kg in 500 mL D5W, infused over 4h, followed by 100 mg/kg in 1000 mL of D5W over next 16h. Filter solution through 0.22 micron filter prior to administration. Complete all 17 doses, even after acetaminophen level falls below critical value.
   -Phytonadione 5 mg IV/IM/SQ (if INR increased).
   -Fresh frozen plasma 2-4 U (if INR increased).
   -Trimethobenzamide (Tigan) 100-200 mg IM/PR q6h prn nausea
10. **Extras:** ECG. Nephrology consult for possible hemodialysis or charcoal hemoperfusion. GI consult.
11. **Labs:** CBC, SMA 7&12, LFT's, INR/PTT, acetaminophen level now & in 4h (plot on nomogram). UA.
12. **Other Orders and Meds:**

THEOPHYLLINE OVERDOSE

1. **Admit to:** Medical intensive care unit.
2. **Diagnosis:** Theophylline overdose
3. **Condition:**
4. **Vital signs:** Neurochecks; Call physician if: BP >160/90, <90/60; P >130; <50; R >25, <10.
5. **Activity:** Bed rest
6. **Nursing:** ECG monitoring until level <20 mcg/mL, aspiration & seizure precautions. Insert single lumen NG tube and lavage with normal saline if recent ingestion.
7. **Diet:** NPO
8. **IV Fluids:** D5½ NS at 125 cc/h
9. **Special Medications:**
   -Activated Charcoal 50 gm PO q4-6h, with sorbitol cathartic (30 mLs of 70% sln) regardless of time of ingestion, until theophylline level <20 mcg/mL. Maintain head-of-bed at 30-45 degrees to prevent aspiration of charcoal.
   -Charcoal hemoperfusion is indicated if serum level >60 mcg/mL, or signs of neurotoxicity, seizure, coma.

Seizure (support oxygenation & respirations): Phenobarbital or lorazepam, see page 77.

10. **Extras:** ECG.
11. **Labs:** CBC, SMA 7 & 12, theophylline level now & in 4h; INR/PTT, liver panel. UA.
12. **Other Orders and Meds:**

TRICYCLIC ANTIDEPRESSANT OVERDOSE

1. **Admit to:** Medical Intensive care unit.
2. **Diagnosis:** TCA Overdose
3. **Condition:**
4. **Vital Signs:** Neurochecks q1h.
5. **Activity:** Bedrest.
6. **Nursing:** Continuous suicide observation. ECG monitoring, measure QRS width, I&O, aspiration and seizure precautions. Place single lumen nasogastric tube and lavage with saline if recent ingestion.
7. **Diet:** NPO
8. **IV Fluids:** NS at 100-150 cc/hr.
9. **Special Medications:**
   -Activated charcoal premixed with Sorbitol 50 gms via NG tube q4-6h round-the-clock until TCA level decreases to therapeutic range. Maintain head-of-bed at 30-45 degree angle to prevent charcoal

aspiration.

-Magnesium citrate 300 mLs via nasogastric tube x 1 dose.

10. **Cardiac Toxicity:** Alkalinization is a cardioprotective measure and has no influence on drug elimination. Treatment goal is to achieve an arterial pH of 7.50-7.55.

-If mechanical ventilation is necessary, hyperventilate to maintain desired pH.

-Administer sodium bicarbonate 50-100 mEq (1-2 amps or 1-2 mEq/kg) IV over 5-10 min, followed by infusion of sodium bicarbonate 2 amps in D5W 1 L at 100-150 cc/h. Adjust rate to maintain pH 7.50-7.55.

11. **Extras:** ECG.

12. **Labs:** Urine toxicology screen, serum TCA levels, liver panel, CBC, SMA-7 & 12, UA.

13. **Other Orders and Meds:**

NEUROLOGY

ISCHEMIC STROKE

1. **Admit to:**
2. **Diagnosis:** Ischemic stroke
3. **Condition:**
4. **Vital signs:** q1-4h with neurochecks; call physician if BP >200/110, <90/60; P >120, <50; R>25, <10; T >38.5°C; or change in neurologic status.
5. **Activity:** Bedrest for 24 hours, then up with assistance and in chair tid if tolerated.
6. **Nursing:** head-of-bed at 30 degrees, turn q2h when awake, range of motion exercises qid, Foley catheter, eggcrate mattress, sheepskin blanket on bed; heal & elbow pads. Guaiac stools, I&O's.
7. **Diet:** NPO until swallowing ability confirmed or dysphagia ground with thickened liquids.
8. **IV Fluids:** LR at 30-100 cc/h.
9. **Special Medications:**

Completed Ischemic Stroke:
   - Aspirin enteric coated 325 mg PO qd **OR**
   - Ticlopidine (Ticlid) 250 mg PO bid.

Cardiogenic, Evolving, or Vertebrobasilar Ischemic Stroke:
   - Heparin, start immediately without bolus in non-hemorrhagic, small to moderate size infarcts: 700-800 U/h (12 U/kg/h) IV (25,000 U in 500 mL D5W); adjust q6-12h until PTT 1.2-1.4 x control.
   - Warfarin 5.0-7.5 mg PO qd x 3d, then 2-4 mg (2-15 mg/d) PO qd. Maintain International Normalizing Ratio of 2-3 Maintain warfarin for patients with evidence of cardiogenic or vertebrobasilar sources).

10. **Symptomatic Medications:**
   - Docusate sodium (Colace) 100 mg PO qhs.
   - Milk of magnesia 30 mL PO qd prn constipation **OR**
   - Bisacodyl (Dulcolax) 10-15 mg PO qhs or 10 mg PR prn.
   - Ranitidine (Zantac) 50 mg IV q6-8h or 150 mg PO bid **OR**
   - Acetaminophen 1-2 tabs PO/PR q4-6h prn temp > 100 or headache.

11. **Extras:** CXR, ECG, CT without contrast or MRI with or without gadolinium; carotid duplex scan; echocardiogram; swallowing studies. Physical therapy consult for passive and active range of motion exercises; neurology, rehab medicine consults.

12. **Labs:** CBC, glucose, SMA 7 & 12, fasting lipid profile, VDRL, ESR; drug levels, INR/PTT, UA. Thrombosis panel, lupus anticoagulant, and anticardiolipin antibody.

13. **Other Orders and Meds:**

TRANSIENT ISCHEMIC ATTACK

1. **Admit to:**
2. **Diagnosis:** Transient ischemic attack
3. **Condition:**
4. **Vital signs:** q1-4h with neurochecks; Call physician if BP >160/90, <90/60; P >120, <50; R>25, <10; T >38.5°C; or change in neurologic status.
5. **Activity:** Up in chair tid if tolerated.
6. **Nursing:** Guaiac stools.
7. **Diet:** Dysphagia ground with thickened liquids or NPO.
8. **IV Fluids:** Heplock with flush q shift.
9. **Special Medications:**
   -Aspirin 325 mg PO qd **OR**
   -Ticlopidine (Ticlid) 250 mg PO bid **OR**
   -Heparin (only if recurrent TIA's; cardiogenic or vertebrobasilar source for emboli), 700-800 U/h (12 U/kg/h) IV infusion, without bolus (25,000 U in 500 mL D5W); adjust q6-12h until PTT 1.2-1.3 x control.
   -Warfarin (Coumadin) 5.0-7.5 mg PO qd x 3d, then 2-4 mg PO qd. Maintain INR of 2.0-3; maintain warfarin for patients with evidence of cardiogenic or vertebrobasilar sources.
10. **Symptomatic Medications:**
    -Docusate sodium (Colace) 100 mg PO qhs.
    -Milk of magnesia 30 mL PO qd prn constipation
    -Ranitidine (Zantac) 150 mg PO bid.
11. **Extras:** CXR, ECG, CT without contrast; carotid duplex scan, echocardiogram. Physical therapy, neurology consults.
12. **Labs:** CBC, glucose, SMA 7 & 12, fasting lipid profile, VDRL, drug levels, INR/PTT, UA. Thrombosis panel, lupus anticoagulant, and anticardiolipin antibody.
13. **Other Orders and Meds:**

SUBARACHNOID HEMORRHAGE

Treatment:
- Stat neurosurgery consult.
- Head of bed at 20 degrees, turn patient q2h, range of motion exercises qid, Foley catheter, eggcrate mattress, heal & elbow pads. Guaiac stools.
- Keep room dark and quiet; no rectal exams; strict bedrest. Neurologic checks q1h for 12 hours, then q2h for 12 hours, then q4h; call physician if abrupt change in neurologic status.
- Diet: Restrict total fluids to 1000 mL/day; remainder of diet as tolerated (if possible, should he high-residue with prunes).
- Nimodipine (Nimotop) 60 mg PO or via NG tube q4h x 21d, must start within 96 hours (not useful in subarachnoid hemorrhage due to trauma).
- Propranolol 1-3 mg IV q6h or 10-60 mg PO qid, titrate to BP <160/90, hold if hypotensive or bradycardic; propranolol-LA (Inderal-LA), 80-120 mg PO qd [60, 80, 120, 160 mg] **OR**
- Nitroprusside sodium, 0.1-0.5 mcg/kg/min (50-200 mg/250 mL NS), titrate to control blood pressure.
- Phenytoin (if seizure) IV load 15 mg/kg IV in NS (infuse at max 50 mg/min) in <u>dextrose free</u> IV, then 300 mg PO/IV qAM (4-6 mg/kg/d).
- Codeine 30-60 mg PO, IM, IV, or SQ q4-6h prn head pain.

Extras: CXR, ECG, CT without contrast; MRI angiogram; cerebral angiogram. Neurology, neurosurgery consults.

Labs: CBC, SMA 7 & 12, VDRL, UA.

Other orders and meds:

INCREASED INTRACRANIAL PRESSURE

Short-Term Measures to Reduce Pressure:
- Stat neurosurgery consult for possible placement ventricular drainage device with monitoring of intracranial pressure, or evacuation of hematoma.
- Restrict fluid to ½ maintenance, isotonic fluids. Head of bed at 30 degrees, head midline.
- Dexamethasone (Decadron) 10 mg IV or IM , followed by 4-6 mg IV, IM or PO q6h.
- Hyperventilation - maintain PCO2 25-30 mm Hg.
- Mannitol, 100 gm (1-1.5 gm/kg) IV over 10-20 min (100 gm in 500 cc D5W), repeated q4-6h as needed; in less severe situations give 37.5-50 gm IV (0.5-1 gm/kg); keep osmolarity <315; do not give for more than 48h.
- Furosemide (Lasix) 40-80 mg IV or PO qd-bid.
- Glycerol 1 gm/kg IV q6h.

-Pentobarbital (barbiturate coma) 7.5 mg/kg/h IV for 3 h, then 2-3 mg/kg/h IV infusion, maintain pentobarbital level of 25-40 mg/L; requires intubation.
Other orders and meds:

SEIZURE & STATUS EPILEPTICUS

1. **Admit to:**
2. **Diagnosis:** Seizure
3. **Condition:**
4. **Vital signs:** q1-4h with neurochecks; Call physician if BP >160/90, <90/60; P >120, <50; R>25, <10; T >38.5°C; or any change in neurological status.
5. **Activity:** Bed rest
6. **Nursing:** Finger stick glucose. Seizure precautions with bed rails up, padded tongue blade at bedside. EEG monitoring. Observe patient as frequently as possible.
7. **Diet:** NPO x 24h, then regular diet if alert.
8. **IV Fluids:** D5½NS at 100 cc/hr; change to hep-lock when taking PO.
9. **Special Medications:**
STATUS EPILEPTICUS
1. Maintain airway.
2. The patient should be positioned laterally with the head down, in order to promote drainage of secretions and prevent aspiration. The head and extremities should be cushioned to prevent injury.
3. During the tonic portion of the seizure, the teeth are tightly clenched. During the clonic phase that follows, however, a bite block or other soft object should be inserted into the mouth to prevent injury to the tongue.
4. 100% O2 by mask, obtain brief history & physical, fingerstick glucose.
5. Secure IV access and draw blood for serum glucose analysis. Give **glucose, 50 mL of 50%** (1 amp) IV (in children, 4 mL/kg of 25% dextrose). Give **thiamine**, 50 mg IV.
6. **Initial Control:**
   Lorazepam (Ativan) 4-8 mg (0.1 mg/kg; not to exceed 2 mg/min) IV at 1-2 mg/min. May repeat 4-8 mg q5-10min (max 80 mg/24h) **OR**
   Diazepam, 5-20 mg slow IV at 1-2 mg/min. Repeat 5-10 mg q5-10 min prn (max 100 mg/24h).
7. **Definitive Seizure Control:**
   Phenytoin 15-20 mg/kg load, in NS at 50 mg/min. Repeat 100-150 mg IV q30min, max 1.5 gms; monitor BP & ECG (QT interval). Hypotension may occur but should not preclude phenytoin; reduce the rate.
   If Seizures Persist, Intubate Patient, Administer Phenobarbital 120-260 mg (10-20 mg/kg) IV at 50 mg/min, repeat 20 mg/kg q15min; additional phenobarbital may be given, up to max of 30-60 mg/kg.

8. **If Seizures Persist, Consider:** Induction of Coma: Pentobarbital 10-15 mg/kg IV over 1-2h, then 1-1.5 mg/kg/h continuous infusion.
9. **Consider Intubation and General Anesthesia**

Maintenance Therapy of Epilepsy:
Primary Generalized:
  First Line Therapy:
    -Carbamazepine (Tegretol) 200-400 mg PO tid [100, 200 mg]. Pre-treatment blood counts, then weekly for 6 weeks, then monthly indefinitely.
    -Phenytoin (Dilantin) loading dose of 400 mg followed by 300 mg q4h x 2 doses (total of 1 g), then 300 mg qd or 100 mg tid or 200 mg bid [30, 50, 100 mg].
    -Valproic acid (Depakene) 250-500 mg PO tid-qid [250 mg].
    -Divalproex (Depakote) 15-30 mg/kg/d PO [125, 250, 500 mg]; less GI irritation than valproic acid.
  Second Line Therapy:
    -Phenobarbital 30-120 mg PO bid [8, 16, 32, 65, 100 mg].
    -Primidone (Mysoline) 250-500 mg PO tid [50, 250 mg]; metabolized to Phenobarbital.
    -Felbamate (Felbatol) 1200-2400 mg PO qd in 3-4 divided doses, max 3600 mg/d [400,600 mg; 600 mg/5 mL susp]; adjunct therapy; high incidence of aplastic anemia.
    -Gabapentin (Neurontin), 300-400 mg PO bid-tid; max 1800 mg/day [100, 300, 400 mg]; adjunct therapy.
    -Lamotrigine (Lamictal) 50 mg PO qd initially, then 50-250 mg PO bid [25, 100, 150, 200 mg]; adjunct therapy .
Partial Seizure:
    -Carbamazepine (Tegretol) 200-400 mg PO tid [100, 200 mg].
    -Valproic acid (Depakene) 250-500 mg PO tid-qid [250 mg].
    -Divalproex (Depakote) 15-30 mg/kg/d PO [125, 250, 500 mg]; less GI irritation than valproic acid.
    -Phenytoin 300 mg PO qd or 200 mg PO bid [30, 50, 100].
    -Phenobarbital 30-120 mg PO tid or qd [8, 16, 32, 65, 100 mg].
    -Primidone (Mysoline) 250-500 mg PO tid [50, 250 mg]; metabolized to phenobarbital.
    -Felbamate (Felbatol) 1200-2400 mg PO qd in 3-4 divided doses, max 3600 mg/d [400,600 mg; 600 mg/5 mL susp]; adjunct therapy; high incidence of aplastic anemia; high incidence of aplastic anemia.
    -Gabapentin (Neurontin), 300-400 mg PO bid-tid; max 1800 mg/day [100, 300, 400 mg]; adjunct therapy.
    -Lamotrigine (Lamictal) 50 mg PO qd initially, then 50-250 mg PO bid [25, 100, 150, 200 mg]; adjunct therapy .

Absence (Petit Mal):

-Ethosuximide (Zarontin) 250-500 mg PO tid-qid [250 mg].

-Valproate 250-500 mg PO tid-qid [250 mg].

-Divalproex (Depakote) 15-30 mg/kg/d PO [125, 250, 500 mg].

-Clonazepam (Klonopin) 0.5-5 mg PO bid-qid [0.5, 1, 2 mg].

-Lamotrigine (Lamictal) 50 mg PO qd initially, then 50-250 mg PO bid [25, 100, 150, 200 mg]; adjunct therapy .

Atypical Absence, Myoclonic:

-Valproate 250-500 mg PO tid-qid [250 mg]; high GI irritation.

-Divalproex (Depakote) 15-30 mg/kg/d PO [125, 250, 500 mg]. Less GI irritation.

-Clonazepam (Klonopin) 0.5-5 mg PO bid-qid [0.5, 1, 2 mg].

-Gabapentin (Neurontin), 300-400 mg PO bid-tid; max 1800 mg/day [100, 300, 400 mg].

10. Extras: MRI with & without gadolinium or CT; EEG (with photic stimulation, hyperventilation, sleep deprivation, awake and asleep tracings); portable CXR, ECG.

11. Labs: CBC, SMA 7, glucose, Mg, calcium, phosphate, liver panel; blood alcohol; ammonia levels, VDRL, anticonvulsant levels. UA, drug screen.

12. Other Orders and Meds:

_____

ENDOCRINOLOGY

DIABETIC KETOACIDOSIS

1. **Admit to:**
2. **Diagnosis:** Diabetic ketoacidosis
3. **Condition:**
4. **Vital signs:** q1h, postural BP & pulse; Call physician if BP >160/90, <90/60; P >140, <50; R >30, <10; T >38.5°C; or urine output < 20 mL/hr for more than 2 hours.
5. **Activity:** Bed rest with bedside commode.
6. **Nursing:** Daily weights, I&O. Foley to closed drainage. Record labs on flow sheet.
7. **Diet:** NPO for 12 hours, then clear liquids as tolerated. Tomorrow begin 1500 calorie American Diabetic Association diabetic diet.
8. **IV Fluids:**

0.5-5 L NS over 1-5h (≥16 gauge), infuse at 400-1000 mL/h until hemo-dynamically stable, then change to 0.45% saline at 150-400 cc/hr; keep urine output > 30-60 mL/h.

Add KCL when no ECG signs of hyperkalemia (peaked T) & urine output adequate, serum K+ ≤ 5.8 mEq/L.

      Concentration.......20-40 mEq KCL/L

      Rate.....................10-40 mEq KCL/hr

May use K phosphate, 20-40 mEq/L, in place of KCL if low phosphate.

Change to **D5** 0.45% saline with 20-40 mEq KCL or K phosphate per liter when blood glucose 250-300.

9. **Special Medications:**

-Oxygen at 2-5 L/min by NC.

-Insulin Regular (Humulin) 7-10 units (0.1 U/kg) IV bolus, then 7-10 U/h IV infusion (0.1 U/kg/h) (50 U in 250 mL of 0.9% saline at 35 mL/hr) (flush IV tubing with 20 mL of insulin sln before starting infusion). Adjust insulin infusion to decrease serum glucose by 100 mg/dL or less per hour.

-After 2 hr of therapy, if bicarbonate level not rising and anion gap not falling, double insulin infusion rate; when bicarbonate level >16 mEq/L and anion gap <16 mEq/L, decrease insulin infusion rate by half

-When the glucose level reaches 250 mg/dL, 5% dextrose should be added to the replacement fluids with KCL 20-40 mEq/L.

-Use 10% glucose at 50-100 mL/h if anion gap still present, & serum glucose <100 mg/dL while on insulin infusion.

-Change to subcutaneous insulin when anion gap cleared; discontinue insulin drip only 1-2h after subcutaneous dose.

10. **Extras:** Portable CXR, ECG.
11. **Labs:** Fingerstick glucose q1-2h. SMA 7 q4-6h. SMA 12, pH, bicarbonate, phosphate, amylase, lipase, hemoglobin A1c; CBC, blood and sputum C&S x

2. Consider cardiac enzymes. UA, urine C&S, serum pregnancy test.
12. Other Orders and Meds:

NONKETOTIC HYPEROSMOLAR SYNDROME

1. **Admit to:**
2. **Diagnosis:** Nonketotic hyperosmolar syndrome
3. **Condition:**
4. **Vital signs:** q1h; Call physician if BP >160/90, <90/60; P >140, <50; R>25, <10; T >38.5°C; or urine output < 20 cc/hr for more than 4 hours.
5. **Activity:** Bed rest with bedside commode.
6. **Nursing** Strict input and output measurement. Foley to closed drainage. Record labs on flow sheet.
7. **Diet:** NPO.
8. **IV Fluids:**
1-5 L NS over 1-6h (≥ 16 gauge IV catheter) until no longer hypovolemic, then give 0.45% saline at 200-300 cc/hr. Maintain urine output ≥ 50 mL/h.
Add 20-40 mEq/L KCL when urine output adequate.
9. **Special Medications:**
   -Insulin Regular 3-5 U/h IV infusion (50 U in 250 mL of 0.9% saline at 15-25 mL/hr).
   -Ranitidine (Zantac) 50 mg IV q6-8h or 150 mg PO bid.
10. **Extras:** Portable CXR, ECG.
11. **Labs:** Fingerstick glucose q1h x 6h, then q6h. SMA 7, osmolality. SMA 12, phosphate, ketones, hemoglobin A1C, CBC, blood and sputum C&S x 2. UA, urine C&S.
12. Other Orders and Meds:

THYROTOXICOSIS & HYPERTHYROIDISM

1. **Admit to:**
2. **Diagnosis:** Thyrotoxicosis
3. **Condition:**
4. **Vital signs:** q1-4h; Call physician if BP >160/90, <90/60; P >130, <50; R>25, <10; T >38.5°C
5. **Activity:** Bed rest
6. **Nursing:** Cooling blanket prn temp >39°C, I&O. Oxygen 2-4 L/min by nasal canula.
7. **Diet:** Regular
8. **IV Fluids:** D5½ NS with 20 mEq KCL at 125 cc/h.

9. Special Medications:

Thyrotoxicosis & Hyperthyroidism:

-Propylthiouracil 300-400 mg PO, then 50-250 mg PO q4-8h, up to 1200 mg/d, usual maintenance dose 50 mg PO tid **OR**

-Methimazole (Tapazole) 30-60 mg PO, then maintenance of 15 mg PO qd-bid **AND**

-Sodium iodide solution (Lugol's solution), 2-6 drops tid for ten days (presurgical preparation and for thyrotoxicosis) **AND**

-Propranolol-LA (Inderal-LA), 80-120 mg PO qd [60, 80, 120, 160 mg]; propranolol 10-40 mg PO q6h or 0.5-1 mg/min, max 2-10 mg IV q3-4h; propranolol decreases heart rate and also decreases the rate of conversion of T3 to the active form, T4 **AND**

-Hydrocortisone IV 100 mg/L q6h.

-Multivitamin tablet PO qd.

-Acetaminophen (Tylenol) 1-2 tabs PO q4-6h prn temp >38°C.

-Triazolam (Halcion) 0.125-0.5 mg PO qhs prn sleep **OR**

-Lorazepam (Ativan) 1-2 mg IV/IM/PO q4-8h prn anxiety or nervousness.

10. Extras: CXR PA & LAT, ECG, endocrine consult. If visual symptoms, obtain ophthalmology consult (rule out exophthalmos and/or optic neuropathy).

11. Labs: CBC, SMA 7&12; sensitive TSH, free T4. UA

12. Other Orders and Meds:

MYXEDEMA COMA & HYPOTHYROIDISM

1. Admit to:

2. Diagnosis: Myxedema Coma

3. Condition:

4. Vital signs: q1h; Call physician if BP systolic >160/90, <90/60; P >130, <50; R>25, <10; T >38.5°C

5. Activity: Bed rest

6. Nursing: Triple blankets prn temp <36°C, I&O, aspiration precautions.

7. Diet: NPO

8. IV Fluids: IV D5 NS with 20 mEq KCL/L at 100-300 cc/hr.

9. Special Medications:

Myxedema Coma & Hypothyroidism:

-Volume replacement with NS at 200-300 cc/h & vasopressors if hypotensive. Correct hypoglycemia with 50% dextrose.

-Levothyroxine (Synthroid, T4, L-Thyroxine) 200-500 mcg IV over 2-4 min, then 100-200 mcg PO or IV qd.

-Hydrocortisone 100 mg IV loading dose, then 50-100 mg IV q8h.

Hypothyroidism in Medically Stable Patient:

-Levothyroxine (Synthroid, T4) 25-50 mcg PO qd, increase by 25-50 mcg PO qd at 2-4 week intervals, to 50-200 mcg qd until TSH normalized. Initial dose 12.5 mcg PO qd if cardiac disease.

11. Extras: ECG, endocrine consult.

12. Labs: CBC, SMA 7&12; sensitive TSH, free T4. UA.

13. Other Orders and Meds:

NEPHROLOGY

RENAL FAILURE

1. **Admit to:**
2. **Diagnosis:** Renal Failure
3. **Condition:**
4. **Vital signs:** tid, postural vitals qAM; Call physician if QRS complex > 0.14 sec; urine output <20 cc/hr; BP >160/90, <90/60; P >120, <50; R>25, <10; T >38.5°C
5. **Allergies:** Avoid magnesium containing antacids, salt substitutes, NSAIDS, & other nephrotoxins. Discontinue phosphate or potassium supplements unless depleted.
6. **Activity:** Bed rest.
7. **Nursing:** Daily weights, I&O, chart urine output q2h; if no urine output for 4h, I&O cath or Foley; Guaiac stools.
8. **Diet:** Renal diet of high biologic value protein of 0.6 to 0.8 g/kg, sodium 2 g, potassium 1 mEq/kg, and at least 35 kcal/kg of nonprotein calories .In oliguric patients, daily fluid intake should be restricted to less than 1 L.
9. **IV Fluids:** D5W at TKO.
10. **Special Medications:**
    -Consider fluid challenge (to rule out pre-renal azotemia if not fluid overloaded) with 500-1000 mL NS IV over 30-60 min. In acute renal failure, I&O cath & check postvoid residual to rule out obstruction.
    -Consider administering diuretics only after adequate central volume has been attained.
    -Furosemide (Lasix) 80-320 mg IV bolus over 10-60 min, double the dose if no response in 2h to total max 1000 mg/24h or furosemide 1000 mg in 250 mLs D5W at 20-40 mg/hr continuous IV infusion **OR**
    -Bumetanide (Bumex) 1-2 mg IV bolus over 1-20 min; double the dose if no response in 1-2 h to total max 10 mg/day.
    -Metolazone (Zaroxolyn) 5-10 mg PO (max 20 mg/24h) **OR**
    -Ethacrynic acid (Edecrin) 50-100 mg IV over 30 min.
    -Mannitol, 12.5-25 gm IV push over 10-20 min, repeated q4-6h as needed; may worsen pulmonary edema if oliguria persists.
    -Dopamine (Intropin) 1-3 mcg/kg per minute IV.
    -Mild hyperkalemia may be treated with sodium polystyrene sulfonate (Kayexalate), 15-30 g orally every 4-6 hours. See page 121.
    -Hyperphosphatemia can be controlled with aluminum hydroxide (Amphojel) 5-10 mL or 1-2 tablets PO given with meals tid.
    -Metabolic acidosis may be treated with sodium bicarbonate to maintain the serum pH >7.2 and the bicarbonate level ≥20 mEq/L. 44-132 mEq (1-3 amps of 7.5%) IV over 5 min, repeat in 10-15 min. Followed by infusion of 2-3 amps in 500 cc of D5W, titrated over 2-4 h.

-Discontinue potentially nephrotoxic meds; aminoglycosides, NSAIDS, sulfonamides, cisplatin, cyclosporine, amphotericin. Adjust all meds to creatinine clearance, & remove potassium from IV.

11. Extras: CXR, ECG, renal ultrasound, Hippurate or technetium renal scan, nephrology & dietetics consults.

12. Labs: CBC, platelets, SMA 7 & 12, potassium, magnesium, phosphate, calcium, uric acid, osmolality, BUN. ESR, INR/PTT. ANA.
Urine specific gravity, UA with micro, urine C&S; 1st AM spot urine electrolytes, creatinine, pH, osmolality, urea; Wright's stain, eosinophiles, electrophoresis. 24h urine protein, creatinine, sodium.

13. Other Orders and Meds:

NEPHROLITHIASIS

1. **Admit to:**
2. **Diagnosis:** Nephrolithiasis
3. **Condition:**
4. **Vital signs:** q shift; Call physician if urine output <30 cc/hr; BP >160/90, <90/60; T >38.5°C
5. **Activity:** Bed rest with bedside commode.
6. **Nursing:** Strain urine, measure inputs and outputs. Place Foley, if no urine for 2 hours.
7. **Diet:** Regular, push oral fluids.
8. **IV Fluids:** IV D5½NS at 100-200 cc/hr (maintain urine output of 80 mL/h).
9. **Special Medications:**
   -Cefazolin (Ancef) 1-2 gm IV q8h
10. **Symptomatic Medications:**
   -Meperidine (Demerol) 75-100 mg & hydroxyzine 25 mg IM q2-4h prn pain **OR**
   -Hydrocodone/Acetaminophen (Vicodin), 1-2 tab q4-6h PO prn pain **OR**
   -Hydromorphone HCL (Dilaudid) 2-4 mg PO q4-6h prn pain **OR**
   -Acetaminophen with codeine (Tylenol 3) 1-2 tabs PO q3-4h prn pain.
   -Zolpidem (Ambien) 10 mg PO qhs.

Note: If stone <5 mm without sepsis then discharge home with analgesics and increase PO fluids. If stone >10 mm and/or fever or increased WBC or signs of ureteral dilation, then consider admission of patient with urology consult.

11. Extras: IVP, KUB, CXR, ECG.

12. Labs: CBC, SMA 6 & 12, calcium, uric acid, phosphorous, UA with micro, urine C&S, urine pH, INR/PTT. Urine cystine (nitroprusside test), send stones for X-ray crystallography. If increased calcium, then check PTH level. 24 hour urine collection for uric acid, calcium, creatinine.

13. Other Orders and Meds:

HYPERCALCEMIA

1. **Admit to:**
2. **Diagnosis:** Hypercalcemia
3. **Condition:**
4. **Vital signs:** q4h; Call physician if BP >160/90, <90/60; P >120, <50; R>25, <10; T >38.5°C; or tetany or any abnormal mental status.
5. **Activity:** Ambulate as often as possible, in chair at other times.
6. **Nursing:** Seizure precautions, weigh patient bid, I & O.
7. **Diet:** Hypercalcemia - restrict calcium to 400 mg/d, push PO fluids.
8. **Special Medications:**
   - -1-4 L of 0.9 % saline over 1-4 hours, then 150-200 cc/h IV until no longer hypotensive **THEN**
   - -Saline diuresis 0.9% or 0.45% saline infused at 150-200 cc/h to replace urine loss **AND**
   - -Furosemide (Lasix) 20-80 mg IV q4-12h. Maintain urine output of 200 mL/h; monitor I & O, monitor serum Na, K+, Mg.
   - -Discontinue medication associated with increased calcium: Thiazide diuretics, lithium carbonate.
9. **Extras:** CXR, ECG, mammogram.
10. **Labs:** Total & ionized calcium, SMA 7 & 12, phosphate, Mg, alkaline phosphatase, prostate specific antigen. 24h urine calcium, potassium, phosphate. Parathyroid hormone.
11. **Other Orders and Meds:**

HYPOCALCEMIA

1. **Admit to:**
2. **Diagnosis:** Hypocalcemia
3. **Condition:**
4. **Vital signs:** q4h; Call physician if BP >160/90, <90/60; P >120, <50; R>25, <10; T >38.5°C; or any abnormal mental status.
5. **Activity:** Up ad lib
6. **Nursing:** I & O.
7. **Diet:** No added salt diet.

8. Special Medications:
Symptomatic HYPOcalcemia:
-Calcium chloride, 10% (270 mg calcium/10 mL vial) give 5-10 mL slowly
over 5-10 min or dilute in 50-100 mL of D5 & infuse over 20 min, repeat
q1-2h if symptomatic, or q6-12h if asymptomatic. Correct hyperphosphatemia before hypocalcemia **OR**
-Calcium gluconate, 20 mL of 10% solution IV (2 vials)(90 mg elemental
calcium/10 mL vial) infused over 10-15min, repeat q1-2h if symptomatic
or q6-12h if asymptomatic **OR** infuse 1 vial in 500 mL of NS IV over 8h

Chronic HYPOcalcemia:
-Calcium carbonate (Oscal) 1 tab PO tid **OR**
-Calcium citrate (Citracal) 1 tab PO q8h.
-Vitamin D2 (Ergocalciferol) 1 tab PO qd.
-Docusate sodium (Colace) 250 mg PO bid prn constipation.

9. Extras: CXR, ECG.
10. Labs: SMA 7 & 12, phosphate, Mg. 24h urine calcium, potassium, phosphate, magnesium.
11. Other Orders and Meds:

HYPERKALEMIA

1. **Admit to:**
2. **Diagnosis:** Hyperkalemia
3. **Condition:**
4. **Vital signs:** Vitals, urine output q4h; Call physician if QRS complex >0.14
sec or BP >160/90, <90/60; P >120, <50; R>25, <10; T >38.5°C.
5. **Activity:** Bed rest; up in chair as tolerated.
6. **Nursing:** I&O, daily weights. Chart QRS complex width q1h.
7. **Diet:** Regular, no salt substitutes.
8. **IV Fluids:** D5NS at 150 cc/h
9. **Special Medications:**
-Consider discontinuing NSAIDS, ACE inhibitors, beta-blockers, K-sparing
diuretics.
-Calcium gluconate 10% sln 10-30 mL IV over 2-5 min; second dose may be
given in 5 min. Contraindicated if digoxin toxicity is suspected. Keep 10
mL vial of calcium gluconate at bedside for emergent use.
-Sodium Bicarbonate 1-3 amps of 7.5% (44-132 mEq) IV over 5 min (give
after calcium in separate IV), repeat in 10-15 min. Follow with infusion of
2-3 amps in 500 cc of D5W, titrated over 2-4 h.
-Insulin 10-20 U regular in 500 mL of 10% dextrose water IV over 1 hr or 10
units IV push with 1 amp 50% glucose (25 gm) over 5 min, repeat as
needed.

-Kayexalate 15-50 gm in 100 mL of 20% sorbitol solution PO now & in 3-4h; up to 4-5 doses/d.

-Kayexalate retention enema 25-50 gm in 200 mL of 20% sorbitol; retain for 30-60 min.

-Furosemide 40-80 mg IV qd-bid.

-Consider emergent dialysis if cardiac complications or renal failure.

10. Extras: ECG

11. Labs: CBC, platelets, SMA7, Mg, calcium, SMA-12. UA, specific gravity, Na, K. pH, 24h urine K, Na, creatinine.

12. Other Orders and Meds:

HYPOKALEMIA

1. **Admit to:**
2. **Diagnosis:** Hypokalemia
3. **Condition:**
4. **Vital signs:** Vitals, urine output q4h; Call physician if BP >160/90, <90/60; P>120, <50; R>25, <10; T >38.5°C.
5. **Activity:** Bed rest; up in chair as tolerated.
6. **Nursing:** I&O
7. **Diet:** Regular
8. **Special Medications:**

HYPOkalemia

-KCL 10-40 mEq in 100 cc saline infused IVPB over 2 hours; or add up to 10-80 mEq to 1 liter of IV fluid and infuse over 2 hours); may combine with 30-40 mEq PO q4h in addition to IV; total dose max is generally 100-200 mEq/d (3 mEq/kg/d).

Chronic Therapy:

-KCL elixir 1-3 tablespoon qd-tid PO after meals (20 mEq/Tbsp of 10% sln).

-Micro-K 10 mEq tabs 2-3 tabs PO tid after meals (40-100 mEq/d).

HYPOkalemia with metabolic acidosis:

-Potassium citrate 15-30 mL in juice qid PO after meals (1 mEq/mL).

-Potassium gluconate 15 mL in juice qid PO after meals (20 mEq/15 mL).

9. **Extras:** ECG, dietetics consult.

10. **Labs:** CBC, SMA7, SMA 12. UA, urine Na, K, Cl, pH, 24h urine for K, Na, creatinine.

11. **Other Orders and Meds:**

HYPERMAGNESEMIA

1. **Admit to:**
2. **Diagnosis:** Hypermagnesemia
3. **Condition:**
4. **Vital signs:** q6h; Call physician if QRS >0.14 sec.
5. **Activity:** Up ad lib
6. **Nursing:** I&O, daily weights. Hold all magnesium containing medications, including antacids if hypermagnesemia.
7. **Diet:** Regular
8. **Special Medications:**
   -Saline diuresis 0.9% or 0.45% saline infused at 100-300 cc/h to replace urine loss **AND**
   -Calcium chloride, 1-3 gms added to saline infusate (10% sln; 1 gm per 10 mL amp) to run at 1 gm/hr **AND**
   -Furosemide 20-40 mg IV q4-6h. Monitor I&O q4-6h, serum Ca, Na, K, Mg bid.
   -Magnesium of >9.0 requires stat hemodialysis (risk for cardiac arrest).
9. **Extras:** ECG
10. **Labs:** Magnesium, calcium, SMA 7 & 12. Urine Mg, electrolytes, 24h urine for Mg, creatinine.
11. **Other Orders and Meds:**

HYPOMAGNESEMIA

1. **Admit to:**
2. **Diagnosis:** Hypomagnesemia
3. **Condition:**
4. **Vital signs:** q6h
5. **Activity:** Up ad lib
6. **Diet:** Regular
7. **Special Medications:**
   -Magnesium sulfate 1-6 gm in 500 mL D5W IV at 1 gm/hr. Hold if no patellar reflex. (Estimation of Mg deficit = 0.2 x kg weight x desired increase in Mg concentration; give deficit over 2-3d) **OR**
   -Magnesium sulfate (severe hypomagnesemia <1.0) 1-2 gm (2-4 mL of 50% sln) IV over 15 min, **OR**
   -Magnesium chloride (Slow-Mag) 65-130 mg (1-2 tabs) PO tid-qid (64 mg or 5.3 mEq/tab) **OR**
   -Milk of magnesia 5 mL PO qd-qid.
   -**Medications Associated with Hypomagnesemia:** Loop diuretics, aminoglycosides, amphotericin, cisplatin.

8. Extras: ECG
9. Labs: Magnesium, calcium, SMA 7 & 12. Urine Mg, electrolytes, 24h urine Mg, creatinine.
10. Other Orders and Meds:

HYPERNATREMIA

1. **Admit to:**
2. **Diagnosis:** Hypernatremia
3. **Condition:**
4. **Vital signs:** q2-4h; Call physician if BP >160/90, <70/50; P >140, <50; R>25, <10; T >38.5°C; or any change in neurologic status.
5. **Activity:** Bed rest; up in chair as tolerated.
6. **Nursing:** I&O, daily weights.
7. **Diet:** No added salt
8. **Special Medications:**

HYPERnatremia:

If volume depleted, give 0.5-3 L NS IV at over 1-3 hours until not orthostatic, then give D5W (if hyperosmolar) or D5½NS (if not hyperosmolar) IV or PO to replace half of body water deficit over first 24h (attempt to correct sodium at 1 mEq/L/h), then remaining deficit over next 1-2 days.

Body water deficit (L) = $\dfrac{0.6(\text{weight kg})([\text{Na serum}]-140)}{140}$

HYPERnatremia with ECF volume excess:

-Salt poor albumin (25%) 50-100 mLs bid-tid x 48-72 h (if low oncotic pressure).
-Furosemide 40-80 mg IV or PO qd-bid.

HYPERnatremia with Diabetes Insipidus:

-D5W to correct body water deficit (see above).
-Pitressin 5-10 U IM/IV q3-4h, keep urine specific gravity ≥1.010 **OR**
-Desmopressin (DDAVP) 1-3 drops intranasal bid (10-20 mcg/d), keep urine SG >1.010

9. **Extras:** CXR, ECG.
10. **Labs:** SMA 7 & 12, osmolality, liver panel, ADH, plasma renin activity. UA, urine specific gravity. Urine Na, K; 24h urine Na, K, creatinine.
11. **Other Orders and Meds:**

HYPONATREMIA

1. **Admit to:**
2. **Diagnosis:** Hyponatremia
3. **Condition:**
4. **Vital signs:** q4h; Call physician if BP >160/90, <70/50; P >140, <50; R>25, <10; T >38.5°C; or any change in neurologic status.
5. **Activity:** Bed rest; up in chair as tolerated.
6. **Nursing:** Seizure precautions, I&O, daily weights.
7. **Diet:** Regular diet.
8. **Special Medications:**

HYPOnatremia with Hypervolemia & Edema (low osmolality <280, UNa <10 mMol/L: nephrosis, CHF, cirrhosis):
-Water restrict to 0.5-1.0 L/d.
-Furosemide 40-80 mg IV or PO qd-bid.

HYPOnatremia with Normal Volume Status (low osmolality <280, UNa <10 mMol: water intoxication; UNa >20: SIADH, hypothyroidism, renal failure, Addison's disease, Stress, Drugs):
-Water restrict to 0.5-1.5 L/d.

HYPOnatremia with Hypovolemia (low osmolality <280) UNa <10 mMol/L: vomiting, diarrhea, 3rd space/respiratory/skin loss; UNa >20 mMol/L: diuretics, renal injury, RTA, adrenal insufficiency, partial obstruction, salt wasting:
  If volume depleted, give 0.5-3 L of 0.9% saline over 1-3 hours until no longer hypotensive, then 0.9% saline at 65-150 cc/h (determine volume as below) or 100-500 cc 3 % hypertonic saline over 5h.

Severe Symptomatic HYPOnatremia:
  If volume depleted, give 0.5-3 L of 0.9% saline (154 mEq/L) over 1-3 hours until no longer orthostatic.
  Determine vol of 3% hypertonic saline (513 mEq/L) to be infused:

  Na (mEq) deficit = 0.6 x (wt kg)x(desired [Na] - actual [Na])

$$\frac{\text{Volume of sln (L)}}{\text{Number of hrs}} = \frac{\text{Sodium to be infused (mEq)}}{\text{(mEq/L in sln) x Number of hrs}}$$

  Correct half of sodium deficit IV slowly over 24 hours until serum sodium is 120 mEq/L; increase sodium by 12-20 mEq/L over 24h (1 mEq/L/h).
-Alternative Method: 3% saline 100-300 cc over 4-6h repeat as needed.
9. **Extras:** CXR, ECG, head/chest CT scan.
10. **Labs:** SMA 7 & 12, osmolality, triglyceride, liver panel. UA, urine specific gravity. Urine osmolality, Na, K.
11. **Other Orders and Meds:**

HYPERPHOSPHATEMIA

1. Admit to:

2. Diagnosis: Hyperphosphatemia

3. Condition:

4. Vital signs: qid

5. Activity: Up ad lib

6. Nursing: I&O

7. Diet: Restrict phosphorus to 0.7-1 gm/d

8. IV Fluids: see below.

9. Special Medications:

Moderate HYPERphosphatemia:

-Aluminum hydroxide (Amphojel) 5-10 mL or 1-2 tablets PO before meals tid

　OR

-Aluminum carbonate (Basaljel) 5-10 mL or 1-2 tablets PO before meals tid.

Severe HYPERphosphatemia:

-Volume expansion with 0.9% saline 1-3 L over 1-3h.

-Acetazolamide (Diamox) 500 mg PO or IV q6h.

-Consider dialysis.

10. Extras: CXR PA & LAT, ECG.

11. Labs: Phosphate, SMA 7 & 12, Mg, Cal, urine electrolytes, pH. UA.

12. Other Orders and Meds:

HYPOPHOSPHATEMIA

1. Admit to:

2. Diagnosis: Hypophosphatemia

3. Condition:

4. Vital signs: qid

5. Activity: Up ad lib

6. Nursing: I&O.

7. Diet: Regular diet.

8. IV Fluids: see below.

9. Special Medications:

Mild HYPOphosphatemia:

-Na or K phosphate 0.25 mMoles/kg in 150-250 mLs D5W or NS, IV infusion over 4h **OR**

-Neutral phosphate (Nutra-Phos), 2 tab PO bid-tid (250 mg elemental phosphorus/tab) **OR**

-Phospho-Soda 5 mL (129 mg phosphorus)PO bid-tid.

Severe HYPOphosphatemia:

-Na or K phosphate 0.5 mMoles/kg in 250 mLs D5W or NS, IV infusion at 10 mMoles/hr.

-Add potassium phosphate to IV solution in place of KCL (max 40 mEq/L infused at 100-150 mL/h); max IV dose 7.5 mg phosphorus/kg/6-8h.

10. Extras: CXR PA & LAT, ECG.

11. Labs: Phosphate, SMA 7 & 12, Mg, Cal, urine electrolytes, pH. UA.

12. Other Orders and Meds:

RHEUMATOLOGY

SYSTEMIC LUPUS ERYTHEMATOSUS

1. **Admit to:**
2. **Diagnosis:** Systemic Lupus Erythematosus
3. **Condition:**
4. **Vital signs:** tid
5. **Allergies:**
6. **Activity:** Up as tolerated with bathroom privileges
7. **Nursing:** Dipstick urine.
8. **Diet:** No added salt, low psoralen diet.
9. **Special Medications:**
   -Aspirin 650-1300 mg PO qid (3.6-5.4 gm/d in divided doses) **OR**
   -Ibuprofen (Motrin) 400 mg PO qid (max 2.4 g/d) **OR**
   -Indomethacin (Indocin) 25-50 mg tid-qid.
   -Hydroxychloroquine (Plaquenil) 200-600 mg/d PO
   -Prednisone 60-100 mg PO qd, may increase to 200-300 mg/d. Maintenance
      10-20 mg PO qd or 20-40 mg PO qOD **OR**
   -Methylprednisolone (pulse therapy) 500 mg IV over 30 min q12h for 3-5d,
      then prednisone 50 mg PO bid.
   -Betamethasone dipropionate (Diprolene) 0.05% ointment applied bid.
   -Ranitidine (Zantac) 150 mg PO bid.
10. **Extras:** CXR PA, LAT, ECG, intermediate strength PPD with controls before starting steroids; echocardiogram. Rheumatology consult.
11. **Labs:** CBC, platelets, SMA 7 & 12. INR/PTT. ESR, complement CH-50, C3, C4, C-reactive protein, LE prep, Coomb's test, VDRL, rheumatoid factor, ANA, DNA binding, lupus anticoagulant, anticardiolipin, antinuclear cytoplasmic; quantitative immunoglobulins; blood cultures x 2. UA, urine culture.
12. **Other Orders and Meds:**

ACUTE GOUT ATTACK

1. **Admit to:**
2. **Diagnosis:** Acute gout attack
3. **Condition:**
4. **Vital signs:** qid
5. **Activity:** Bed rest with bedside commode
6. **Nursing:** Keep foot elevated with support sheets over foot; guaiac stools.
7. **Diet:** Low purine diet.
8. **Special Medications:**
   -Indomethacin (Indocin) 50 mg PO q6h x 2d, then 50 mg tid for 2 days, then 25 mg PO tid **OR**
   -Ketorolac (Toradol) 30-60 mg IM, then 15-30 mg IM q6h or 10 mg PO tid-qid. **OR**
   -Ibuprofen (Motrin) 800 mg, then 400-800 mg PO q4-6h **OR**
   -Naproxen sodium (Anaprox, Anaprox-DS) 550 mg PO bid.
   -Colchicine 2 tablets (0.5 mg or 0.6 mg) followed by 1 tablet q1h until relief, max dose of 9.6 mg/24h. Then give maintenance colchicine 0.5-0.6 mg PO qd-bid **OR**
   -Methylprednisolone (SoluMedrol) 125 mg IV x 1 dose **THEN**
   -Prednisone 40-60 mg PO qd x 5 days, followed by tapering.
   -Intra-articular injection with lidocaine/marcaine and triamcinolone.

Hypouricemic Therapy:
   -Hypouricemic drugs are contraindicated during an acute attack unless patient was previously taking them.
   -Allopurinol 300 mg PO qd, may increase by 100-300 mg q2weeks.
   -Probenecid (Benemid), 250 mg bid. Increase the dosage to 500 mg bid after 1 week, then increase by 500-mg increments every 4 weeks while monitoring the serum uric acid level, which should be maintained below 6.5 mg/dL. Max dose 2 g/d; average maintenance dosage is 500 mg bid.

9. **Symptomatic Medications:**
   -Ranitidine (Zantac) 150 mg PO bid.
   -Meperidine (Demerol) 50-100 mg IM/IV q4-6h prn pain.
10. **Labs:** CBC, SMA 7, uric acid, ESR. UA with micro. Synovial fluid for light and polarizing micrography for crystals; C&S, Gram stain, glucose, protein, cell count, pH. X-ray views of joint. 24 hour urine for uric acid, creatinine.
11. **Other Orders and Meds:**

FORMULAS

A-a gradient = $[(P_B - PH_2O) FiO_2 - PCO_2/R] - PO_2$ arterial

$$= (713 \times FiO2 - pCO2/0.8) - pO2 \text{ arterial}$$

P_B = 760 mmHg; PH_2O = 47 mmHg; R ≈ 0.8
normal Aa gradient <10-15 mmHg (room air)

Arterial oxygen capacity = (Hgb(gm)/100 mL) x 1.36 mL O2/gm Hgb

Arterial O2 content = 1.36(Hgb)(SaO2)+0.003(PaO2)= NL 20 vol%

O2 delivery = CO x arterial O2 content = NL 640-1000 mL O2/min

Cardiac output = HR x stroke volume

$$CO \text{ L/min} = \frac{125 \text{ mL O2/min/M}^2}{8.5\{(1.36)(Hgb)(SaO2) - (1.36)(Hgb)(SvO2)\}} \times 100$$

Normal CO = 4-6 L/min

Na (mEq) deficit = 0.6 x (wt kg) x (desired [Na] - actual [Na])

$$SVR = \frac{MAP - CVP}{CO_{L/min}} \times 80 = \text{NL 800-1200 dyne/sec/cm}^2$$

$$PVR = \frac{PA - PCWP}{CO_{L/min}} \times 80 = \text{NL 45-120 dyne/sec/cm}^2$$

$$GFR \text{ mL/min} = \frac{(140 - age) \times wt \text{ in kg}}{72 \text{ (males) x serum creatinine (mg/dL)}}$$
85 (females) x serum creatinine (mg/dL)

$$\text{Creatinine clearance} = \frac{U \text{ creatinine (mg/100 mL)} \times U \text{ vol (mL)}}{P \text{ creatinine (mg/100 mL)} \times \text{time (1440 min for 24h)}}$$

Normal creatinine clearance = 100-125 mL/min(males), 85-105(females)

$$\text{Body water deficit (L)} = \frac{0.6(\text{weight kg})([\text{measured serum Na}]-140)}{140}$$

$$\text{Serum Osmolality} = 2 [Na] + \frac{BUN}{2.8} + \frac{Glucose}{18} = 270-290$$

Na (mEq) deficit = 0.6 x (wt kg)x(desired [Na] - actual [Na])

$$\text{Fractional excreted Na} = \frac{U \text{ Na/ Serum Na}}{U \text{ creatinine/ Serum creatinine}} \times 100 = \text{NL<1\%}$$

Anion Gap = Na + K - (Cl + HCO3)

For each 100 mg/dL ↑ in glucose, Na+ ↓ by 1.6 mEq/L.

Corrected = measured Ca mg/dL + 0.8 x (4 - albumin g/dL)
serum Ca$^+$ (mg/dL)

Ideal body weight males = 50 kg for first 5 feet of height + 2.3 kg for each additional inch.

Ideal body weight females = 45.5 kg for first 5 feet + 2.3 kg for each additional inch.

Basal energy expenditure (BEE):
Males=66 + (13.7 x actual weight Kg) + (5 x height cm)-(6.8 x age)
Females= 655+(9.6 x actual weight Kg)+(1.7 x height cm)-(4.7 x age)

Nitrogen Balance = Gm protein intake/6.25 - urine urea nitrogen - (3-4 gm/d insensible loss)

Predicted Maximal Heart Rate = 220 - age

Normal ECG Intervals (sec)
PR	0.12-0.20
QRS	0.06-0.08

Heart rate/min	Q-T
60	0.33-0.43
70	0.31-0.41
80	0.29-0.38
90	0.28-0.36
100	0.27-0.35

DRUG LEVELS OF COMMON MEDICATIONS

DRUG	THERAPEUTIC RANGE*
Amikacin	Peak 25-30; trough <10 mcg/mL
Amitriptyline	100-250 ng/mL
Carbamazepine	4-10 mcg/mL
Chloramphenicol	Peak 10-15; trough <5 mcg/mL
Desipramine	150-300 ng/mL
Digitoxin	10-30 ng/mL
Digoxin	0.8-2.0 ng/mL
Disopyramide	2-5 mcg/mL
Doxepin	75-200 ng/mL
Ethosuximide	40-100 mcg/mL
Flecainide	0.2-1.0 mcg/mL
Gentamicin	Peak 6.0-8.0; trough <2.0 mcg/mL
Imipramine	150-300 ng/mL
Lidocaine	2-5 mcg/mL
Lithium	0.5-1.4 mEq/L
Nortriptyline	50-150 ng/mL
Phenobarbital	10-30 mcg/mL
Phenytoin**	8-20 mcg/mL
Procainamide	4.0-8.0 mcg/mL
Quinidine	2.5-5.0 mcg/mL
Salicylate	15-25 mg/dL
Streptomycin	Peak 10-20; trough <5 mcg/mL
Theophylline	8-20 mcg/mL
Tocainide	4-10 mcg/mL
Valproic acid	50-100 mcg/mL
Vancomycin	Peak 30-40; trough <10 mcg/mL

* The therapeutic range of some drugs may vary depending on the reference lab used.
** Therapeutic range of phenytoin is 4-10 mcg/mL in presence of significant azotemia and/or hypoalbuminemia.

COMMONLY USED ABBREVIATIONS

1/2NS	0.45% saline solution	CPK	creatinine phosphokinase
a.c.	ante cibum (before meals)		
ABG	arterial blood gas	CPK-MB	myocardial-specific CPK isoenzyme
ac	before meals		
ACTH	adrenocorticotropic hormone	CPR	cardiopulmonary resuscitation
ad	right ear		
ad lib	ad libitum (as needed or desired)	CSF	cerebrospinal fluid
		CT	computerized tomography
ADH	antidiuretic hormone		
AFB	acid-fast bacillus	CVA	cerebrovascular accident
alk phos	alkaline phosphatase		
ALT	alanine aminotransferase	CVP	central venous pressure
am	morning		
AMA.	against medical advice	CXR	chest x-ray
amp	ampule	d/c	discharge; discontinue
amt	amount	D5W	5% dextrose water solution; also D10W, D50W
AMV	assisted mandatory ventilation; assist mode ventilation		
ANA	antinuclear antibody	DIC	disseminated intravascular coagulation
ante	before		
AP	anteroposterior		
aq	water	diff	differential count
ARDS	adult respiratory distress syndrome	dil	dilute
		DKA	diabetic ketoacidosis
as, al	left ear	dL	deciliter
ASA	acetylsalicylic acid	DOSS	docusate sodium sulfosuccinate--a stool softener
AST	aspartate aminotransferase		
au	both ears		
bid	bis in die (twice a day)	DT's	delirium tremens
B-12	vitamin B-12 (cyanocobalamin)	ECG	electrocardiogram
BM	bowel movement	ER	emergency room
BP	blood pressure	ERCP	endoscopic retrograde cholangiopancreatography
BUN	blood urea nitrogen		
c/o	complaint of		
c̄	cum (with)	ESR	erythrocyte sedimentation rate
C and S	culture and sensitivity		
C	centigrade	ET	endotracheal tube
C3, C4	third and fourth complement components	ETOH	alcohol
		F	Fahrenheit
Ca	calcium	Fe/TIBC	iron/total iron-binding capacity
cap	capsule		
CBC	complete blood count; includes hemoglobin, hematocrit, red blood cell indices, white blood cell count, and platelets	Fe	iron
		FEV_1	forced expiratory volume (in one second)
cc	cubic centimeter	FiO2	fractional inspired oxygen
CCU	coronary care unit		
cm	centimeter	fl	fluid
CMF	cyclophosphamide, methotrexate, and fluorouracil	g	gram(s)
		GC	gonococcal; gonococcus
CNS	central nervous system		
CO_2	carbon dioxide	GFR	glomerular filtration rate
COPD	chronic obstructive pulmonary disease		
		GI	gastrointestinal

gm	gram	MI	myocardial infarction
gt	drop	MIC	minimum inhibitory concentration
gtt	drops		
h .hr	hour	mL	milliliter
H20	water	mm	millimeter
HBsAG	hepatitis B surface antigen	MOM	Milk of Magnesia
HCO3	bicarbonate	MRI	magnetic resonance imaging
Hct	hematocrit		
HDL	high-density lipoprotein	Na	sodium
Hg	mercury	NaHCO3	sodium bicarbonate
Hgb	hemoglobin concentration	Neuro	neurologic
HIV	human immunodeficiency virus	NG	nasogastric
hr	hour	NKA	no known allergies
hs	hora somni (bedtime, hour of sleep)	NPH	neutral protamine Hagedorn (insulin)
IM	intramuscular	NPO	nulla per os (nothing by mouth)
I & 0	intake and output-- measurement of the patient's intake by any route (mouth, intravenous, rectum) and output by any route, including urine, vomit, diarrhea, and fluid from bleeding or drainage	NS	normal saline solution (0.9%)
		NSAID	nonsteroidal anti-inflammatory drug
		O2	oxygen
IU	international units	OD	right eye
ICU	intensive care unit	oint	ointment
IgM	immunoglobulin M	OS	left eye
IMV	intermittent mandatory ventilation	Osm	osmolality
		OT	occupational therapy
INH	isoniazid	OTC	over the counter
IPPB	intermittent positive-pressure breathing	OU	each eye
		oz	ounce
IV	intravenous or intravenously	p, post	after
IVP	intravenous pyelogram; intravenous piggyback	p.c.	post cibum (after meals)
K, K+	potassium	PA	posteroanterior; pulmonary artery
kcal	kilocalorie		
KCL	potassium chloride	PaO2	arterial oxygen pressure
KPO4	potassium phosphate		
KUB	x-ray of abdomen (kidneys, ureters, bowels)	pAO2	partial pressure of oxygen in alveolar gas
L	liter		
LDH	lactate dehydrogenase	PB	phenobarbital
LDL	low-density lipoprotein	pc	after meals
liq	liquid	pCO2	partial pressure of carbon dioxide
LLQ	left lower quadrant		
LP	lumbar puncture, low potency	PEEP	positive end-expiratory pressure
LR	lactated Ringer's (solution)		
MB	myocardial band	per	by
MBC	minimal bacterial concentration	pH	hydrogen ion concentration (H +)
		PID	pelvic inflammatory disease
mcg	microgram		
mEq	milliequivalent	pm	afternoon
mg	milligram	PO	orally
Mg	magnesium	PO	per os (by mouth)
Mg	magnesium	pO2	partial pressure of oxygen
MgSO4	Magnesium Sulfate		

Abbreviation	Definition
polys	polymorphonuclear leukocytes
PPD	purified protein derivative
PR	per rectum
prn	as needed
prn	pro re nata (as needed)
Pro	prothrombin
PT	physical therapy; prothrombin time
PTCA	percutaneous transluminal coronary angioplasty
PTT	partial thromboplastin time
PVC	premature ventricular contraction
q	quaque (every) q6h, q2h every 6 hours; every 2 hours
qid	quarter in die (four times a day)
qAM	every morning
qd	quaque die (every day)
qh	every hour
qhs	every night before bedtime
qid	4 times a day
qOD	every other day
qs	quantity sufficient
R/O	rule out
RA	rheumatoid arthritis; room air; right atrial
Resp	respiratory rate
RL	Ringer's lactated solution (also LR)
ROM	range of motion
rt.	right
s	sine (without)
s/p	status post (the condition of being after)
sat	saturated
SBP	systolic blood pressure
SC	subcutaneousiy
SGOT	serum glutamic-oxaloacetic transaminase (AST)
SGPT	serum glutamic-pyruvic transaminase (ALT)
SIADH	syndrome of inappropriate antidiuretic hormone
SL	sublingually under tongue
SLE	systemic lupus erythematosus
SMA-12	sequential multiple analysis; a panel of 12 chemistry tests performed together on a 12-channel autoanalyzer. Tests generally include Na⁺, K⁺, HCO3 , Chloride , BUN, glucose, creatinine, bilirubin, calcium, total protein, albumin, and alkaline phosphatase. Other chemistry panels include SMA-6 and SMA-20
SMX	sulfamethoxazole
sob	shortness of breath
sol	solution
SQ	under the skin
ss	one-half
STAT	statim (immediately)
susp	suspension
t.i.d.	ter in die (three times a day)
T4, T3RU	thyroxine level (T4) and triiodothyronine resin uptake
tab	tablet
TB	tuberculosis
Tbsp	tablespoon
Temp	temperature
TIA	transient ischemic attack
tid	three times a day
TKO	to keep open, an infusion rate (usually 500 mL/24h)--just enough to keep the IV from clotting
TMP	trimethoprim
TMP-SMX	trimethoprim-sulfamethoxazole combination
TPA	tissue plasminogen activator
TSH	thyroid-stimulating hormone
tsp	teaspoon
U	units
UA	urinalysis
ung	ointment
URI	upper respiratory infection
USP	United States Pharmacopeia
Ut Dict	as directed
UTI	urinary tract infection
VAC	vincristine, Adriamycin, and cyclophosphamide
vag	vaginal
VC	vital capacity
VDRL	Venereal Disease Research Laboratory
VF	ventricular function
V fib	ventricular fibrillation
VLDL	very low-density lipoprotein
Vol	volume

CO_2 (note: HCO_3, Na^+, K^+)

VS	vital signs
VT	ventricular tachycardia
W	water
WBC	white blood count
x	times

INDEX

5-aminosalicylate 65
Absence seizure 79
  a fib 57
Accupril 19
Acetaminophen 35, 74, 85
Acetaminophen overdose 71
Acetaminophen/codeine 33, 85
Acetazolamide 92
Acetylcysteine 71
ACLS 6
Actigall 60
Activated charcoal 28, 72
Acute Bronchitis 27
Acyclovir 42, 43
Adenocard 20
Adenosine 20
Aerobid 25
Albumin 90
  colloid 46
Albuterol 25, 26, 29, 41
Alcohol withdrawal 69
Aldactone 58
Allopurinol 95
Alprazolam 70
Alteplase 33
Aluminum carbonate 92
Aluminum hydroxide 84, 92
Alupent 25, 26
Alveolar/arterial O2 gradient 32, 96
Ambien 17, 49, 54, 85
Amikacin 45
Amikin 45
Aminophylline 25, 27, 29
Aminophylline levels 25
Aminosalicylate 65
aminosalicylate enema 65
Aminosyn 66
Amiodarone 22
Amoxicillin 49
Amoxicillin/clavulanate 26, 38, 49, 50
Amphojel 84, 92
Amphotericin B 37, 44
  bladder irrig 50
  fungemia 46
Ampicillin 26, 35, 40, 47-50, 61
Ampicillin/Sulbactam 26, 27, 38, 44, 46
Anaerobic Pneumonia 40
Anaphylaxis 28
Anaprox 95
Anaprox-DS 95
Ancef 49, 51, 53, 85
Angina 16, 18
Anistreplase 16
Antibiotic colitis 63
APSAC 16
Aralen 94
Arfonad 23
Ascites 58
Aspiration Pneumonia 39

Aspirin 16, 75
Asthma 25
Atenolol 17, 22
  MI 17
Ativan 17, 21, 77
Atovaquone 41
Atrovent 27
Augmentin 26, 38, 50
Axid 56
Azactam 49, 53
Azithromycin 38, 40
Azlocillin 40
Azmacort 25, 27
Aztreonam 49, 53
Azulfidine 64, 65
B12 64-66
Bactrim 41, 63
Barbiturate coma 77
Basaljel 92
Beclomethasone 25, 27
Beclovent 25, 27
Benadryl 17, 29, 55, 59, 70
Benazepril 19
Benemid 95
Benzodiazepine overdose 70
Benztropine 70
Berotec 26
Betadine 53
Betamethasone 94
Biaxin 38, 40
Bicarbonate 99
Biliary sepsis 61
Bisacodyl 74
Bitolterol 26
Body water deficit 90, 96
Branhamella catarrhalis 40
Bretylium 21, 22
Brevibloc 17, 21
Budesonide 25
Bumetanide 19, 84
Bumex 19, 84
Calcium carbonate 87
Calcium chloride 87
Calcium citrate 87
Calcium gluconate 87
Campylobacter 63
Candida cystitis 50
Candida septicemia 46
Capoten 19
Captopril 19, 58
Carbamazepine 78, 97
Carbon monoxide 70
Cardioversion 20, 22
Cardizem 21
Catapres 23
Catapres-TTS 23
Ceclor 26, 27
Cefaclor 26
Cefadroxil 49
Cefazolin 49, 51, 53, 85
Cefixime 49
Cefizox 35, 40, 45, 47, 50
Cefonicid 40
Cefotan 54, 60

Cefotaxime 35, 38, 45, 47
Cefotetan 54, 60
Cefoxitin 45, 47, 48, 53, 54, 60-62
Ceftazidime 35, 39, 40, 45, 46, 50, 51, 55
Ceftin 38
Ceftizox 35, 38-40
Ceftizoxime 35, 38, 40, 45, 47, 50
Ceftriaxone 35, 38, 44, 45, 49
  Meningitis 35
  pneumonia 40
Cefuroxime 26, 27, 38, 40
Cefuroxime axetil 38
Cellulitis 53
Central Parenteral Nutrition 66
Cephalothin 49
Cerebral vascular accident 74
Charcoal 28, 70-72
Chenix 57
Chenodiol 60
Chloramphenicol 40, 97
Chlordiazepoxide 69
Chloroquine 94
Cholangitis 61
Cholecystitis 60
Chronic obstruct pulm dis 26
Cimetidine 56, 57, 66
Cipro 44, 48-50, 53, 63
Ciprofloxacin 44, 48-51, 53, 62, 63
Cirrhosis 58
Citracal 87
Claforan 35, 38, 45, 47
Clarithromycin 38, 40
Cleocin 39, 40, 48, 53
Clindamycin 39, 43, 46, 48, 53
Clofazimine 43
Clonazepam 79
Clonidine 23
  HTN crisis 23
  patch 23
Clostridium difficile 63
Clotrimazole 42
Coccidioidomycosis 44
Coccidiomycosis 44
Codeine 76
  antidiarrheal 67
Cogentin 70
Colace 17, 39
Colchicine 95
Compazine 56, 59
Congestive Heart Failure 19
COPD 26
Cordarone 22
Coumadin 32
Cozaar 19
Crohn's disease 64

Cryptococcus neoformans 43
Cryptosporidium 64
CSF 35
Cytomegalovirus 43
Cytovene 43
Dapsone 41
Darvocet 32
DDAVP 90
DDC 41
DDI 41
Decadron 76
Deep vein thrombosis 31
Delirium Tremens 69
Demerol 33, 51, 54
Depakene 78
Depakote 78
Depo-Medrol 29
Desmopressin 90
Dexamethasone 76
Diabetic ketoacidosis 80
Diamox 92
Diarrhea 62, 63
Diazepam 69, 77
    alcohol withdrawals 69
    seizures 77
Dicloxacillin 53
Didanosine 41
Diflucan 42, 44, 50
Digoxin
    psvt 21
Digoxin loading dose 19
Dilantin
    arrhythmia 22
Dilaudid 85
Diltiazem 21
Dimenhydrinate 17
Dipentum 65
Diphenhydramine 16, 17, 29,
    55, 59, 70
Diphenoxylate 63, 67
Diprolene 94
Disopyramide 22
Divalproex 78
Diverticulitis 48
Dobutamine 19, 46
    CHF 19
Docusate 17, 21, 39
Dopamine 46
    CHF 19
Doxycycline 54
Dramamine 17
Dulcolax 74
Duricef 49
Edecrin 84
Edema 58
Enalapril 19, 23
Encephalopathy
    hepatic 68
Endocarditis 36
Entamoeba 63
Enteral feeding 67
Enteroinvasive E coli 63
Enterotoxic E coli 63
Epinephrine 28, 29
Eramycin 38

Ergocalciferol 87
Erythromycin 38, 40, 53, 63
Erythropoietin 42
Esmolol 17, 21, 22
Esophagitis 42
Ethacrynic 84
Ethambutol 43, 52
Ethanol 70
Ethmozine 22
Ethosuximide 79
Ethylene glycol 70
Extrapyramidal reaction 70
Famotidine 56, 57
Felbamate 78
Felbatol 78
Fenoterol 26
Filgrastim 42
Flagyl 40, 53
Flecainide 22
Fleroxacin 62
Floxin 49, 62
Fluconazole 42, 44
    cystitis 50
Flucytosine 47
Fludrocortisone 24
Flumazenil 70
    Romazicon 70
Flunisolide 25, 27
Fluogen 34
Folic acid 33
Fortaz 35, 40, 45, 50, 51
Foscarnet 42
Fosinopril 19
Fresh frozen plasma 71
Fungal Endocarditis 37
Furosemide 89
    ascites 58
    CHF 19
    renal failure 84
G-CSF 42
Gabapentin 78, 79
Ganciclovir 43
Gastric lavage 70
Gentamicin 36, 50
GI bleeding 57
Giardia 64
Giemsa 42
Glycerol 76
Gout 95
Granulocyte colony-
    stimulating factor 42
Haemophilus influenzae 40
Halcion 82
Heart failure 19
Helicobacter pylori 56
Hemodialysis 70
Hemoperfusion 72
Hemoptysis 27
Heparin 17, 31, 32
Heparin overdose 31
Hepatitis 59
Herpes encephalitis 43
Herpes simplex 42
Herpes varicella zoster 43
Hespan 46

Hetastarch 46
Histoplasmosis 44
Hivid 41
Humulin 80
Hydrocodone 85
Hydrocortisone 29, 82
    enema 65
Hydromorphone 85
Hydroxychloroquine 94
Hydroxyzine 33, 85
Hyperbaric oxygen 70
Hypercalcemia 86
Hyperkalemia 87
Hypermagnesemia 89
Hypernatremia 90
Hyperosmolar syn 81
Hyperphosphatemia 92
Hypertensive emergency
    23
Hyperthyroidism 81
Hyperventilation 76
Hypocalcemia 86
Hypokalemia 88
Hypomagnesemia 89
Hyponatremia 91
Hypophosphatemia 92
Hypothyroidism 82
Ibuprofen 94, 95
Imipenem/Cilastatin 39,
    44, 46
Imipenem/cilastatin 39
Imodium 63, 65, 67
Indocin 94
Indomethacin
    gout 95
    sle 94
Influenza vacc 34
INH 43
Insulin 80
    hyperkalemia 87
Intracranial pressure 76
Intralipid 66
Iodoquinol 63
Ipecac 70
Ipratropium 27
Ischemic Stroke 74
Isoniazid 43, 52, 99
Isoproterenol 22, 29
Isoptin 20
Isordil 17, 20
Isosorbide 17, 20
    MI 17
Isospora 64
Isuprel 22, 29
Itraconazole 44
Kaopectate 63, 65, 67
Kayexalate 84, 88
KCl 88
Keflex 49
Ketoconazole 22, 42
Ketorolac 95
Klebsiella pneumoniae 40
L-Thyroxine 82
Labetalol 23
    HTN crisis 23

Lactulose 68
Lamictal 78, 79
Lamotrigine 78, 79
Lamprene 43
Lasix 58, 76, 84, 86
Legionella pneumoniae 40
Leucopenia 42
Leucovorin 43
Levophed 29
Levothyroxine 82
Librium 69
Lidocaine 21, 22
Lisinopril 19
   CHF 19
Lomefloxacin 49
Lomotil 63, 67
Loperamide 63, 65, 67
Lopressor 17
Lorazepam 17, 21, 77
Losartan 19
Lotensin 19
Lugol's solution 82
Macrodantin 49
Magnesium 89
Magnesium citrate 70, 73
Magnesium deficit 89
Magnesium sulfate 22, 70, 89, 99
Mannitol 76, 84
Maxair 26
Maxaquin 49
Mefoxin 45, 47, 48, 51, 53, 54, 60-62
Meningitis 35
Meperidine 33, 49, 51, 52, 54, 56
Mepron 41
Mesalamine 65
Methanol 70
Methimazole 82
Methylprednisolone 16, 25, 27, 29, 33, 41, 65, 94, 95
   asthma 25
   enema 65
   sle 94
Methylprednisolone acetate 29
Metoclopramide 67, 69
Metolazone 19, 58, 84
   CHF 19, 58
Metronidazole 40, 46-48, 53, 56, 63, 64, 68
Metroprolol 17
Mexiletine 22
Mexitil 22
Mezlocillin 40, 45, 46, 55, 60, 61
Micro-K 88
Midazolam 20
Milk of magnesia 74, 75, 89
Milrinone 19
Monocid 40
Monopril 19
Moraxella 40

Moraxella catarrhalis 40
Morcizine 22
Morphine 33
Motrin 94, 95
Mucomyst 71
Mycelex 42
Mycobacterium Avium Complex 43
Mycobutin 44
Mycoplasma pneumoniae 40
Mycostatin 42
Myocardial infarction 16
Mysoline 78
Myxedema coma 82
Nafcillin 36, 40, 51, 53
Naloxone 70
Naproxen 95
Naproxen sodium 95
Naproxen sodium 95
Narcan 70
Narcotic overdose 70
Neomycin 68
Nephrolithiasis 85
Nephrology 84
Neupogen 42
Neurontin 78, 79
Neutropenia 42
Neutropenia/Gancyclovir- Induced leucopenia 42
Neutropenic fever 54
Nifedipine 23
   HTN crisis 23
Nimodipene 76
Nimotop 76
Nitrofurantoin 49
Nitroglycerin
   HTN crisis 23
Nitroglycerine 16, 20
   CHF 20
   MI 16
Nitroprusside 23, 76
Nizatidine 56
Nizoral 42
Nonketotic hyperosmolar syn 81
Nonketotic hyperosmolar syn 81
Norepinephrine 29
Norfloxacin 49, 50, 62
Noroxin 49, 50, 62
Nutra-Phos 92
Nystatin 42
Octreotide 63
Oflox 63
Ofloxacin 62, 63
Olsalazine 65
Oncologic emergency 54
Opportunistic infections AIDS 42
Oral Candidiasis 42
Oscal, 87
Osmolality, estimate of 96
Osmolite 67
Osteomyelitis 51

Oxacillin 36, 40, 51, 53
Pancreatitis 61
Paracentesis 48, 58, 59
Parenteral nutrition 66
Paromomycin 64
Paroxysmal supravent tach 20
PCP prophylaxis 41
Pelvic inflam dis 54
Penicillin 33, 36, 37, 39, 40, 47, 53
Penicillin V 33
Pentam 41
Pentamidine 41
Pentobarbital 78
   coma 77
Pepcid 56, 57
Pepsid 56
Peptic ulcer disease 56
Pepto Bismol 63
Pepto-Bismol 56
Peripheral parenteral supplementation 66
Peritonitis 47
Phenazopyridine 50, 51
Phenobarbital 77, 78
Phenothiazine reaction 70
Phentolamine, 23
Phenytoin 76-78
   arrhythmia 22
pheochromocytoma 23
Phosphate 92, 93
Phospho-Soda 92
Phytonadione 31, 71
Piperacillin 39, 40, 55, 61
Pirbuterol 26
Pitressin 57, 90
Plaquenil 94
Pleural effusion 29
Pleurocentesis 30
Pneumococcal pneumoniae 40
Pneumocystis carinii pneumonia 41
Pneumocystis pneumonia 41
Pneumonia 38, 40
Pneumovax 34
Poisoning 70
Post-exposure Prophylaxis HIV 41
Postural Syncope 24
Potassium 66, 88
   elixir 88
Potassium citrate 88
Potassium gluconate 88
Prednisone 25, 27, 95
   asthma 25
   sle 94
Primacor 19
Primaxin 39, 44, 46, 47
Primidone 78
Prinivil 19
Probenecid 95
Procainamide 21, 22, 97

Valproate 79
Valproic 78
Vancomycin 40, 51, 53, 63
Varicella 43
Vasopressin 57
Vasotec 19, 23
Vasovagal Syncope 24
Ventolin 25, 26, 29
Ventricular arrhythmias 21
Ventricular fibrillation 21
Ventricular tachycardia 21
    Distinguishing from
    SVT 21
Verapamil 20
Versed 20
Vibramycin 54
Vicodin 85
Videx 41
Vistaril 29, 33
Vitamin B12 66
Vitamin B6 43
Vitamin D2 87
Vitamin K 31, 57
Warfarin 31-33, 74, 75
Warfarin overdose 31
Yersinia 63
Zalcitabine 41
Zantac 26, 56, 57, 62
Zarontin 79
Zaroxolyn 19, 58, 84
Zestril 19
Zidovudine 41-43
Zidovudine-Induced
    Neutropenia 42
Zinacef 26, 27, 38, 39
Zithromax 38, 40
Zolpidem 17, 49, 54, 85
Zoster 43
Zovirax 42

Synthroid 82
Systemic lupus 94
T4 82
Tagamet 56, 57, 66
Tambocor 22
Tapazole 82
Tegretol 78
Tenormin 17
Terbutaline 25
Tetracycline 56
Theo-Dur 25
Theophylline 20, 25-27, 29,
    70, 72, 97
    IV 25
Theophylline overdose 72
Thrombolytics 16
Thyrotoxicosis 81
Ticarcillin 39
Ticarcillin/clavulanate 38,
    47, 50
Ticarcillin/clavulanic 44, 46,
    47, 50, 51, 53, 60
Ticlid 75
Ticlopidine 75
Tigan 56, 71
Timentin 38, 44, 46, 47, 50,
    51, 53, 60
Timolol 22
Tinidazole 63
Tissue plasminogen
    activator 17, 33, 100
TMP-SMX 41
TMP/SMX 39, 41
Tobramycin 39, 40, 44-48,
    50, 55
Tocainide 22
Tonocard 22
_oradol 95
_nalate 26
ades de pointes 21
_ology 70
_nsmosis 43
_3
_chemic attack 75
_rhea 63
_25, 27, 95
_ssant

_ne 66
_23
_razine 56, 59
_ne 22
_ne 32
_ne overdose 70
_l 22, 76
_-LA 82
_racil 82
_31
_mbranous colitis
_as aeruginosa 40
_embolism 32
_tis 50
_43, 52
_51
_3
_ne 43
_4
_56, 57, 67

ProCalamine 66
Procardia 23
Prochlorperazine 56, 59
Promix 67
Propafenone 22
Propoxyphene 32
Propoxyphene overdose 70
Propranolol 22, 76
  a fib 21
  MI 17
Propranolol-LA 82
Propylthiouracil 82
Protamine 31
Pseudo-membranous colitis 63
Pseudomonas aeruginosa 40
Pulmonary embolism 32
Pyelonephritis 50
Pyrazinamide 43, 52
Pyridium 50, 51
Pyridoxine 43
Pyrimethamine 43
Quinacrine 64
Quinapril 19
Quinidine 22
Ranitidine 26, 56, 57, 67
Reglan 67, 69
Renal failure 84
Retrovir 41
Rhythmol 22
Rifabutin 44
Rifampin 36, 37, 40, 43, 51, 52
Rocephin 35, 38, 44, 45, 49
Saline diuresis 86, 89
Salmonella 63
Sandostatin 63
Scopolamine 24
Seizure 77
  Absence 79
Septic arthritis 44
Septic shock 45
Septra 27, 38, 41, 49, 50
Shigella 63
SIADH 91, 100
Sickle crisis 33
Slow-Mag 89
Sodium 66
Solu-Medrol 25, 27, 29, 95
Sorbitol 68, 72, 88
Spironolactone 58
Sporanox 44
Staphylococcus aureus 40
Status epilepticus 77
Stool studies 63
Streptokinase 16
Stroke 74
Subarachnoid 76
Sulfadiazine 53
Sulfasalazine 64, 65
Supraventricular Tachycardia
  distinguishing from VT 21
Suprax 49
Syncope 24
Synovial fluid 95

Synthroid 82
Systemic lupus 94
T4 82
Tagamet 56, 57, 66
Tambocor 22
Tapazole 82
Tegretol 78
Tenormin 17
Terbutaline 25
Tetracycline 56
Theo-Dur 25
Theophylline 20, 25-27, 29, 70, 72, 97
  IV 25
Theophylline overdose 72
Thrombolytics 16
Thyrotoxicosis 81
Ticarcillin 39
Ticarcillin/clavulanate 38, 47, 50
Ticarcillin/clavulanic 44, 46, 47, 50, 51, 53, 60
Ticlid 75
Ticlopidine 75
Tigan 56, 71
Timentin 38, 44, 46, 47, 50, 51, 53, 60
Timolol 22
Tinidazole 63
Tissue plasminogen
  activator 17, 33, 100
TMP-SMX 41
TMP/SMX 39, 41
Tobramycin 39, 40, 44-48, 50, 55
Tocainide 22
Tonocard 22
Toradol 95
Tornalate 26
Torsades de pointes 21
Toxicology 70
Toxoplasmosis 43
TPA 17
Trandate 23
Transient ischemic attack 75
Travelers diarrhea 63
Triamcinolone 25, 27, 95
Triazolam 82
Tricyclic Antidepressant
  Overdose 72
Trimethaphan 23
Trimethobenzamide 56, 71
Trimethoprim/SMX 38, 41, 48-50, 63
Tuberculosis 43, 52
  in aids 43
Tylenol 39, 85
Tylenol #4 85
Tylenol 3 33
Ulcerative colitis 65
Unasyn 26, 27, 38, 47
Urinary tract infection 49
Ursodiol 60
Vaginitis 42
Valium 69

Valproate 79
Valproic 78
Vancomycin 40, 51, 53, 63
Varicella 43
Vasopressin 57
Vasotec 19, 23
Vasovagal Syncope 24
Ventolin 25, 26, 29
Ventricular arrhythmias 21
Ventricular fibrillation 21
Ventricular tachycardia 21
  Distinguishing from SVT 21
Verapamil 20
Versed 20
Vibramycin 54
Vicodin 85
Videx 41
Vistaril 29, 33
Vitamin B12 66
Vitamin B6 43
Vitamin D2 87
Vitamin K 31, 57
Warfarin 31-33, 73, 74, 75
Warfarin overdose 31
Yersinia 63
Zalcitabine 41
Zantac 26, 56, 57, 62
Zarontin 79
Zaroxolyn 19, 58, 84
Zestril 19
Zidovudine 41-43
Zidovudine-Induced
  Neutropenia 42
Zinacef 26, 27, 38, 39
Zithromax 38, 40
Zolpidem 17, 49, 54, 85
Zoster 43
Zovirax 42